Praise for An A–Z Guide to Healing Foods

"A Super Guide to Super Foods! 'Let food be thy medicine,' and let Elise Marie Collins be the Hippocrates of healing food guides."
—**Kenneth D. Fine, MD**, founder and director of The Intestinal Health Institute and the EnteroLab.com Reference Laboratory

"The encyclopedic information about the nutritional, medical, and holistic benefits of foods in *An A–Z Guide to Healing Foods* is so fascinating that every time I look something up, I just keep reading. Thanks to Elise Collins, who has made this the easiest shopper's guide ever. I now shop smarter and eat better."
—**Dana Jacobi**, author of *12 Best Foods Cookbook* and *The Essential Best Foods Cookbook*

"As a nutrition doctor, I have dedicated my career to the idea of food as medicine. This book is a wonderful tool for people who also believe in this concept and want to make the best possible and most enjoyable eating choices for optimal health."
—**Melina B. Jampolis, MD**, author of *The No-Time-to-Lose Diet*

"This useful guide reminds us that an amazing array of edibles, from the mundane to the exotic, deserve to be labeled 'superfoods.'"
—**Daphne Miller, MD**, author of *The Jungle Effect*

"This easy-to-use companion belongs in the kitchen for everyday use. Health expert Elise Collins has distilled an enormous amount of information into a compact, concise resource on the nutritional properties and healing benefits of foods. This book brings to your kitchen the practical knowledge of using food as your medicine for healing yourself and your family."
—**Kami McBride**, herbalist

"Straightforward, clear, and organized simply, *An A–Z Guide to Healing Foods* contains lots of information about what is in a wide variety of foods, as well as where to shop for them. I especially like the suggestions for how to use food to spur healing of many common illnesses and problems. Elise Collins has helped simplify the confusion about what to eat by making finding and understanding nutritional facts both fascinating and accessible. Highly recommended for foodies and emerging foodies."

    —**Judith Hanson Lasater, PhD**, yoga teacher since 1971
        and author of 8 books including *Yogabody: Anatomy, Kinesiology and Asana*

An A–Z Guide to Healing Foods

A Shopper's Companion

Elise Marie Collins

Conari Press

First published in 2009 by
Red Wheel/Weiser, LLC
With offices at:
500 Third Street, Suite 230
San Francisco, CA 94107
www.redwheelweiser.com

ISBN: 978-1-57863-419-0
LIBRARY OF CONGRESS CATALOGING-IN-PUBLICATION DATA AVAILABLE UPON REQUEST.

Cover design by Maija Tollefson
Text design by Maxine Ressler
Typeset in Fournier and Super Grotesk A
Cover photographs: Blueberries © kone/iStockphoto.com; cranberries © pederk/ iStockphoto.com; pomegranate © Anna Sedneva/iStockphoto.com; sugar peas © Alisdair James/iStockphoto.com

Printed in Canada
TCP
10 9 8 7 6 5 4 3 2 1

The paper used in this publication meets the minimum requirements of the American National Standard for Information Sciences—Permanence of Paper for Printed Library Materials Z39.48-1992 (R1997).

Contents

Acknowledgments

Thank you to the spirit in each of us that seeks peace, love, and greater good for all. Thank you to Ragi and Krishna for your encouragement, support, and down-to-earth sensibility. Thanks to my parents for their support, especially my mom who always made fresh peas. Thank you to Amber Guetebier, Ali McArt, Jordan Overby, and Jan Johnson of Red Wheel/Weiser and Conari Press. Thank you Yunah Kim and Brenda Knight.

Introduction

Throughout history, cultures have relied on the plants and edibles around them for cures. Before Viagra, the Aztecs believed avocados were potent aphrodisiacs. Ancient Greeks used carrots instead of Zantac to soothe their stomach ailments. Native Americans administered chocolate instead of Tylenol to break a fever. Long before calorie counting, double-blind studies, laboratory studies of edible plant extracts, and other scientific investigations, humans used food to alleviate symptoms, acquire energy, create stamina, uplift the spirit, mend wounds, increase fertility, and much more. Food has always been used as medicine.

Biology and nutritional science have logically explained the process of eating, digesting, and assimilating our diet. Just in the last century, vitamins were discovered and a scientific model of food was born. Food was divided into macronutrients such as proteins, carbohydrates, and fats. Micronutrients like vitamins, minerals, and phytonutrients were studied and categorized. Much has been learned in the era of nutritional labels, but it's important to remember that there is so much more to the healing properties of food and diet. An attitude of reverence for the miraculous alchemy of the human body reminds us to be humble in our present knowledge and to acknowledge that our views of the medicinal value of foods are ever evolving.

Surrounded by processed, junk, and fast foods in grocery stores, on the job, and at the corner café, we are challenged to choose vital, minimally processed, healing foods. This guide strives to inspire through scientific research, ancient wisdom, common sense, and an increasing base of knowledge of therapeutic foods. A few years ago a powerful healing fruit called acai was relatively unknown outside of Brazil, where it's been used medicinally for centuries. Now millions see the health benefits of acai touted everywhere—from *The Oprah Winfrey Show* to the Internet. Let this guide serve to inspire you to explore, prepare, procure, grow, taste, savor, and enjoy healing foods that suit your individual needs. Get ready to fight inflammation with string beans, prevent cancer with broccoli sprouts, and build immunity with shitake mushrooms!

The A–Z Guide

Acai (ah-SAH-ee): Grown mainly in South America, fresh acai berries may be hard to find in Europe or North America. Yet even when consumed frozen, powdered, in a paste, or as a juice, acai has more antioxidants than almost any other food. Acai is an excellent source of potassium, B vitamins, vitamins C and E as well as magnesium, copper, zinc, and phosphorus. Beta-sitosterol, a phytosterol found in acai, has been shown to lower unhealthy LDL cholesterol. Acai juice or smoothies have anti-inflamatory properties and can help reduce symptoms of arthritis. Scientific interest is growing on acai's ability to prevent or help reverse cancer. Lab tests showed that acai berry extract exposed to human leukemia cells killed between 45 and 86 percent of the cancerous cells. Research on this turbocharged antioxidant berry is continuing, but its reputation as an Amazonian superfood precedes it. ↠ *Preparation tip:* Avoid acai processed with high heat.

Acerola: A berry rich in ascorbic acid, acerola is also known as Barbados cherry. Acerola grows on a tropical fruit-bearing shrub in warmer climates, from southern Texas to Mexico and down to South America. Also cultivated in India and highly prized for their potent healing powers, acerola berries are an excellent food-based source of vitamin C, bioflavonoids, rutin, and other vitamin C cofactors. Vitamin C helps build collagen, the stuff of bones, teeth, and connective tissue. And of course it will ward off the common cold. ↠ *Preparation tip:* If you live in Texas or Florida, find acerola berries fresh or grow your own. Otherwise buy acerola dried into powder or made into pills or tablets.

Superfoods

Mother nature made some foods remarkable in their ability to heal and prevent illness. Some of these superfoods have even been known to rival the healing ability of pharmaceutical drugs. Nutrient dense, packed with curing power, vitamins, minerals, and phytonutrients, superfoods are in the eye of the beholder. Anyone can call a food a superfood; there is no certifying government board that bequeaths the title. This subjectivity leads to confusion—what's super for you may not be super for everyone. Superfoods have numerous known vitamins, minerals, and compounds. But many beneficial substances that have not yet been isolated, discovered, or labeled are also likely to be part of superfoods. The synergy between known and unknown compounds, vitamins, and minerals in superfoods is another component of their efficacy. Sometimes scientists are sure a food is helpful for preventing or reversing symptoms of a disease or condition, but they don't know how or why the food is working. Be aware of foods that have been declared superfoods—sometimes it's nothing but marketing hype. Is the term used with integrity, or to promote a product without much substance? The quality of the processing of such declared superfoods, as well as the quantity of the superfoods contained in the packaged product, are critical to that food's ability to heal. Look for superfoods straight from mother nature—like seaweed, fresh turmeric, or blueberries. Or seek out superfoods produced by reputable producers.

Adzuki Beans; Aduki Beans; Azuki Beans: Native to Japan, nutty and sweet adzuki beans are high in protein and plentiful in vitamins and minerals. A favored food in macrobiotic cuisine, adzuki beans are easier to digest than most legumes. Considered the most yang of all beans in macrobiotic cuisine, adzuki beans have plenty of fiber, folic acid and B vitamins, and high levels of trace minerals like molybdenum, copper, manganese, and zinc. Adzuki beans are used to make red bean paste.

Agar; Agar-Agar: Most often used as a vegetarian substitute for gelatin, which is made from animal protein, agar can help fight inflammation and relieve constipation. A great source of calcium and iron, agar can also be added to broths or teas, or used as a thickening agent in sauces or preserves. Made from a red algae called gelidium, agar is very fibrous and, when wet, it triples in size. Agar's expansive properties make those who eat it feel full. It's a popular ingredient in foods promoted for weight loss.

Agave: Considered sacred by the Aztecs, agave comes from a plant indigenous to Central and South America. Agave has a low glycemic index, creating less of a spike in blood sugar levels than most processed sugars. A flavorful amber liquid, similar to a runny honey, agave delivers sweetness without the unpleasant sugar rush that is associated with processed sugar or artificial corn syrup. For these reasons many diabetics have found agave to be a safe alternative to conventional sweeteners or chemical, diet sweeteners. Raw chefs recommend using unheated agave.

Ajwain (AHJ-oh-wen): A staple seed found in Indian kitchens, ajwain contains thymols that are antibacterial and antiseptic. Related to cumin and caraway, ajwain is often used to add flavor to samosas as well as lentil or potato dishes and roasted nuts. Pungent and bitter, ajwain seeds are often chewed after a large meal to aid digestion and freshen breath. Ayurveda recommends carminative ajwain for many gastrointestinal disorders such as lack of appetite, indigestion, flatulence, and diarrhea.

Alfalfa: Alfalfa's unusually deep roots can grow to over fifteen feet, allowing them to pull minerals from deep in the earth's surface. Consequently alfalfa has a naturally high content of essential and nonessential minerals such as calcium, phosphorus, potassium, and iron, all culled from the soil. Plentiful in vitamins and eight essential amino acids, alfalfa has powerful nourishing and rebuilding properties. Alfalfa can help build and purify blood, so it is helpful in treating anemia. It's also known to heal ulcers as well as boost immunity. Great for people who are fearful of green veggies, dried and powdered alfalfa can be added to smoothies, baked goods, and other foods to give them a boost of green power. Pregnant and nursing mothers will find alfalfa provides a great source of much-needed absorbable calcium and minerals. ⇥ *Preparation tip:* Add dried or fresh alfalfa to boiled water for a nutrient-rich tea. As a whole food additive, powdered alfalfa can boost smoothies, juices, and even baked foods.

Alfalfa Sprouts: Pound for pound, alfalfa sprouts rank among the most powerful antioxidant vegetables, surpassed only by kale, brussels sprouts, garlic, and spinach. Sprinkling delicate and sweet alfalfa sprouts on sandwiches, soups, and salads isn't just for hippies; it has been scientifically proven to disarm specific harmful free radicals and hydroxyl and peroxyl radicals. Alfalfa sprouts contain vitamins C, B_2, and B_5 as well as folic acid, copper, molybdenum, zinc, manganese, and magnesium. Food-based phytoestrogens are found in abundance in alfalfa sprouts and are known to be critical factors in the prevention of cancer, osteoporosis, menopausal symptoms, and heart disease. Saponins in alfalfa and especially alfalfa sprouts are beneficial phytochemicals that can lower unhealthy LDL cholesterol without affecting healthy HDL cholesterol. Alfalfa sprouts can be purchased in most grocery or health food stores.

Almond: Considered in Ayurveda to be the most beneficial of all nuts, almonds help build *ojas,* or vital essence. In the Indian science, foods like almonds not only nourish the body, but increase our spiritual and intellectual abilities. Almonds have a high concentration of protein and nutrients and are a good source of vitamin E, calcium, zinc, potassium, magnesium, and iron. Ayurveda recommends peeling or blanching almonds to remove the difficult-to-digest outer skin. Blanch or soak almonds overnight, and then remove the peel by squeezing it off the almond. Soaking raw almonds improves digestibility and nutrient content. Soaking also activates the ability of almonds to take seed, as it starts them sprouting, thereby releasing many nutrients as the almond prepares to transform from seed to plant. Unfortunately most almonds in the United States originate from California and legally must be flash pasteurized, a sterilization method that destroys many vital enzymes and minerals. Raw almonds can only be purchased directly from farmers at farmers markets or imported raw from other countries. Almonds are the only nuts that alkalize the body. Almond milk was commonly used in medieval times when cow's milk was hard to come by. ↠ *Preparation tip:* Enjoy nutritious, dairy-free, fresh almond milk. Soak 1 cup almonds in 4 cups water overnight, place in a blender, blend, strain, and enjoy. Peeling or blanching the almonds is a little more time-consuming, but will makes the almond milk less bitter and more auspicious, according to Ayurveda.

Aloe Vera: Known as the miracle plant, mysterious and alluring aloe vera has been used for centuries for its medicinal properties. Gandhi consumed aloe juice to sustain him during long fasts.

Almost every system of the body benefits from this stupendous superplant. A natural antibacterial, antifungal, and antiviral agent, aloe has been used as a traditional cure for all diseases of the stomach and intestines, including ulcers. From the sixteenth to nineteenth centuries, the internal gel of aloe was processed and used as a commercial laxative. Rich in plant sterols, amino acids, and polysaccharides, aloe is often used as a liver cleanser. Known in Sanskrit by a name that means "goddess," aloe has toning and fortifying properties for women. It helps alleviate menopausal symptoms aggravated by a sluggish liver. Aloe vera juice can help stabilize blood sugar levels and help boost immunity. Externally, aloe vera has been used for wound healing, sunburn alleviation, and as an additive for antiaging creams. Aloe has been shown to improve digestion and assimilation of nutrients in the digestive tract. Commonly used as a detox herb, aloe has a growing reputation as a weight loss aid. Look for minimally processed aloe gel, juice, or canned aloe pieces. To preserve vital phytonutrients, avoid heating aloe products to high temperatures. A natural antibiotic, antibacterial, and antifungal, aloe vera helps a long list of ailments and conditions. Fresh aloe vera leaves can be ordered online or, in the right climate, grown in your yard. ➼ *Preparation tip:* The leaves can be filleted to remove the hard outer coating. The most potent part of the plant is the gel, which can be added to drinks or smoothies. Pregnant or nursing women and children should not consume aloe vera gel, especially fresh gel, because of the cleansing effects on the liver.

Amaranth: A highly nutritious grain revered by the ancient Aztecs, amaranth was used in religious rituals and consumed by Aztec athletes. Ancient Greeks believed that this unique seed bestowed immortality and gave it a name derived from the Greek word *amarantos,* which means "unfading." World health workers discovered that in areas of Africa and Latin America where amaranth grows, there is little or no incidence of malnutrition.

Amaranth thrives in poor soil and in drought conditions, making it a miraculous storehouse of energy and nutrition for people in poor farming regions. Extremely high in protein, vitamin C, calcium and magnesium, iron, lysine, and silicon, amaranth makes a great healing agent. It is an excellent vegetarian food source for infants, children, and nursing and pregnant women, whose calcium, protein, and mineral needs are high. Amaranth also benefits those with hypertension and cardiovascular disease, as regular consumption of the grain has been shown to reduce blood pressure and cholesterol levels. Amaranth appears to lower cholesterol via its content of plant stanols and squalene. A gluten-free, high-fiber grain, amaranth flour can be substituted for healthier baking.

Amaranth greens are super suppliers of B vitamins and minerals including calcium, manganese, potassium, iron, and magnesium. Studies have pointed to amaranth greens, also known as Chinese spinach, as helpful in lowering unhealthy cholesterol. Research suggests that when amaranth greens are consumed, the liver enzyme 7 alpha-hydroxylase significantly increases, which helps to break down cholesterol into bile acids. Numerous other animal studies have verified amaranth green's cholesterol-busting potential. Avoid amaranth greens if you have any type of kidney disorder, as they contain high levels of oxalic acid. →→ *Preparation tip:* Make amaranth breakfast cereal by mixing ½ cup steel-cut oats and ½ cup amaranth with 2½ cups water. Bring to a boil, and then simmer for 15–20 minutes. Steel-cut oats mask amaranth's crunchy consistency.

Amasake: A traditional Japanese sweetening agent made of fermented sweet rice, amasake is often recommended in macrobiotic recipes as a less processed sweetener that is relatively easy to digest. Many health food stores carry *koji*, the beneficial bacterial starter for amasake, or the dark, syrupy liquid sweetener itself.

Amla Berry; Amalaki; Indian Gooseberry: Amla berries have the highest known concentration of natural vitamin C of any food. Amla berries grow on trees in India where they have been used medicinally for thousands of years. In Ayurvedic medicine, amla berries are often consumed in a specially prepared medicinal paste. Before the advent of modern pharmaceuticals, ancient Indian sages blended herbs and foods into pastes and gels. These formulas are still regularly consumed by millions of people in India and around the world to prevent degenerative diseases as well as to alleviate symptoms from many chronic conditions. Chyavanprash is one such formula made mainly of amla berries and can be found in many health food stores. Amla berries also strengthen veins and support the circulatory system. It's highly unlikely that you'll find fresh green, tangy amla berries in the supermarket, but amla paste, juice, powder, or pills are usually available in health food stores.

Anise: Anise is a rich source of coumarin compounds, which have shown potential to prevent cancer. Anise seeds are good for digestion and remedying bad breath. The combination of phytochemicals in anise has a wide range of health benefits, most notably helping the body expel gas and relax intestinal spasms. Anise gives foods a licorice flavor. Some say that anise will cure the hiccups as well. A blend of anise seeds, fennel seeds, sesame seeds, coconut, sugar, and peppermint oil, called *Mukhwas,* is often served after an Indian meal for better digestion and to freshen the breath.

Apple: Apples, like blue jeans, are ubiquitous and sturdy. Apples seem to fit into everyone's dietary wardrobe. They come in many designs or varieties and can be found everywhere from the corner store to the gourmet grocer. One of apples' best health boosting agents is found in its skin—the miraculous antioxidant quercetin has been found to have natural anti-inflammatory and antihistamine properties. Eating apples can help alleviate symptoms of seasonal allergies. Apples also contain vitamin C and a healthy dose of both insoluble and soluble fiber. Consuming apples has been associated with decreased risk of cancer, asthma, heart disease, and type 2 diabetes. An apple a day will help lower cholesterol, lower blood pressure, alleviate symptoms of gout and arthritis, and promote digestive regularity.

Apple Cider Vinegar: Made from fresh fermented apple juice, apple cider vinegar has been used as a folk medicine for countless ailments from acne to indigestion. Preliminary studies on apple cider vinegar and its main ingredient, acetic acid, have evidenced support for these remedies. Studies have shown apple cider vinegar may lower total cholesterol and triglycerides while helping to keep blood sugar levels steady. Many report that drinking a mixture of apple cider vinegar and water helps them keep the pounds away, provides relief from acid reflux, and can be used to treat arthritis and gout. ➻ *Preparation tip:* Drink raw, organic, unfiltered, unpasteurized apple cider vinegar. Make an alkalizing cocktail by mixing 8 ounces of water with two teaspoons of apple cider vinegar. Sip and, if you don't enjoy the flavor, add 1-2 teaspoons of raw honey.

Apricot: A stone fruit, the apricot was brought from China to Greece by Alexander the Great. Hundreds of years later, the first apricot tree was delivered to Virginia in 1720. Apricots are pocket-size, carotenoid-rich secret weapons against macular degeneration, many forms of cancer, and heart disease. Rich in potassium and iron, apricots are as fiber-filled as they are juicy.

Arame: A dark and thick seaweed, arame blends well into soups or salads. Plentiful in iron, protein, calcium, and iodine, arame supports the spleen and pancreas in traditional Chinese medicine. Rich in phytonutrients, arame gets its brown color from a plant compound called fucoxanthin that Japanese researchers have found promotes fat burning in rats. ➻ *Preparation tip:* British nutritionist Dr. Gillian McKeith recommends cooking arame with root vegetables such as turnips and parsnips. *See also* **Seaweed.**

Artichoke; Cardoon: Fresh and festive, artichokes found in markets in the United States are almost always globe artichokes. The hearts and inner leaves of these unusual flowers have a unique, somewhat bitter flavor. High in fiber, vitamins A and C, folic acid, niacin, riboflavin, thiamine, biotin, magnesium, manganese, chromium, and potassium, fresh artichokes are low in calories and fat. Most of the carbohydrates in artichokes come from inulin, an oligosaccharide that is handled differently than other sugars in the body—it can only be partially digested. The undigested portion serves as food for friendly bacteria in the digestive tract, making the artichoke a natural probiotic food. Particularly beneficial to diabetics, inulin in artichokes has been shown to assist in keeping blood sugar levels under control. Traditionally artichokes are known for healing the liver. Silymarin, a compound that helps liver tissue regenerate, can be found in artichokes and milk thistle. Artichokes assist the gallbladder in generating bile and increasing the flow of bile to and from the liver. Artichokes' effects on the liver and gallbladder make them a helpful food for those suffering from hepatitis and other liver diseases. Artichokes have also been used traditionally as a diuretic and to lower blood fats and cholesterol.

Arugula: A sassy, pungent, and bitter green from the mustard family that was considered by ancient Romans and Egyptians to be a potent aphrodisiac, arugula is high in vitamins A and C, niacin and iron, riboflavin, calcium and magnesium, potassium, copper, and zinc-phosphorus. This rich mineral blend makes arugula's ragged leaves an effective alkalizing food, helping balance the diet of someone who eats meats or processed foods or has high levels of stress. Glucosinates in arugula are powerful antioxidants that protect against many forms of cancer. Because the glucosinates stimulate the natural detoxifying enzymes of the body, arugula can help release stored toxins. Greens like arugula contain many phytochemicals, such as carotene and chlorophyll.

Asian Pear: Crisp Asian pears have some vitamin C and fiber and have an especially high water content. *See also* **Pear.**

Top Twelve Most Contaminated Fruits and Vegetables

Peaches	Nectarines	Grapes
Apples	Cherries	Pears
Bell Peppers	Strawberries	Spinach
Celery	Lettuce	Potatoes

Twelve Least-Contaminated Fruits and Vegetables

Asparagus	Cauliflower	Onions
Avocados	Corn	Papaya
Bananas	Kiwi	
Broccoli	Mangoes	

Although washing fruits and vegetables reduces surface residues of harmful chemicals, some pesticides are absorbed directly into the edible portion of the plant. Some chemicals specifically resist removal and are designed to adhere to the surface of the fruit or vegetable. Peeling will remove some pesticides, but you will also lose extremely beneficial nutrients located in the skin of a fruit or vegetable.

Asparagus: Low in calories and high in protein and antioxidants, asparagus contains plenty of potassium; vitamins A, B6, C, and K; folate; riboflavin; and thiamine. Asparagus is also a good source of dietary fiber and niacin. It can help balance your system if you have been overconsuming acidic foods like meat, grains, or junk food. Alkalizing asparagus can also help to alleviate any overly acidic conditions. Folate levels in asparagus are particularly high, making this unique green a great choice for pregnant and nursing mothers. Research suggests that consuming folate benefits those at risk for cardiovascular problems and helps protect against cancer. Traditionally asparagus was used to treat arthritis. Ayurvedic medicine esteems asparagus as an aphrodisiac, kidney strengthener, and overall tonifying food for women.

Avocado: Green and luscious, avocados have surprisingly more protein than any other fruit, about 2 grams per 4-ounce serving. The Aztecs thought avocados were an aphrodisiac. Truly a fruit, avocados are rich in luteins and two notable phytochemicals, one of which, glutathiaone, has demonstrated anticancer properties. Lutein is known for safeguarding against hardening of the arteries and atherosclerosis and for preventing prostate cancer. It also protects the eyes from cataracts and age-related macular degeneration. Avocados are loaded with fat, but it's the kind of fat that heals. Avocados come chock-full of vitamin C, potassium, and folic acid and have the highest soluble fiber of any fruit.

Azomite Powder: A miraculous mineral powder mined from ancient seabeds in Utah, azomite powder is recommended by the Weston A. Price Foundation. Unlike chemically isolated vitamins and supplements, azomite is an edible mineral powder made by Mother Nature. It detoxifies by pulling positively charged pathogens out of the human body and is also sold as a soil amendment.

↠ *Preparation tip:* Azomite powder serves as an excellent source of calcium and magnesium that you can add to smoothies or bake into breads and casseroles.

Bamboo Shoots: Fresh bamboo shoots are an excellent source of thiamine, vitamin B6, and potassium. Canning destroys most vitamins and minerals, but even canned bamboo shoots are low-calorie sources of healthy fiber. ↠ *Preparation tip:* Look for fresh bamboo shoots in Asian markets. Parboil or cook, since uncooked bamboo shoots are toxic.

Banana; Plantain: Bananas are excellent sources of potassium, vitamins B6 and C, riboflavin, magnesium, and biotin. As a plentiful supplier of potassium, one of the most important electrolytes in the body, bananas offer protection against heart disease and strokes. In fact, except for strawberries, bananas are higher in minerals than any other fruit, with 80 mg of silicon, 33 mg of magnesium, and 26 mg of phosphorus as well as trace amounts of copper, chromium, iron, fluoride, manganese, selenium, and zinc per serving. Studies have shown that bananas help children recover from diarrhea. Related to bananas, plantains are commonly eaten as vegetables in African, Caribbean, and Latin American countries. The high fiber content and low sugar of plantains, or *plantanos*, promote healthy digestion. Plantains need to be cooked before eating. ↠ *Preparation tip:* Try sautéing plantains in olive oil or coconut oil or steaming them and serving them mashed with a natural sweetener like agave.

Barley: Barley is a powerful healer for the spleen and pancreas and a regulator of the stomach in traditional Chinese medicine. Known to fortify the intestinal tract, barley can be helpful in treating diarrhea. Roman athletes ate barley for stamina. High in magnesium, selenium, copper, and phosphorous, barley's fiber is also high in beta-glucan. Binding bile acids and ushering them through the digestive tract, beta-glucan helps to lower cholesterol and boost immunity. Whole barley is called sproutable, meaning it will start to grow roots and stems when immersed in water. When sprouted, barley contains twice as much calcium, three times the iron, and 25 percent more protein, magnesium, phosphorus, copper, and chromium, which is critical in helping the body maintain blood glucose levels. Barley contains numerous other healing compounds, including many antioxidants that help reduce the risk of cancer and heart disease. Barley is low in gluten, but not gluten free. One of the most acid-forming grains, barley can be rendered more alkalizing by roasting it until aromatic before cooking. ➤➤ *Preparation tip:* Add barley to vegetable soup to make it heartier and more nutritious. Steep 1 cup of barley with 4 cups of water to make barley water, a healing food tea that can be served hot or cold.

Barley Grass: Grass-fed beef is better for you than corn-fed beef. Why? Grasses like wheat and barley are uniquely suited to nutritionally sustain animals and humans. Anthropologists know that early humans munched on a wide variety of rejuvenating grasses growing on the ancient savannas in Africa. Gluten-free, rich in vital nutrients, enzymes, chlorophyll, and even protein, barley grass contains a powerful antioxidant called superoxide dismutase, or SOD. Like all antioxidants, SOD goes after free radicals, but SOD seems to be particularly effective at attacking destructive molecules formed by exposure to radiation, chemical exposure, or other toxins. Barley grass has plenty of life-affirming qualities: it's oxygenating, alkalizing, and easily digestible. Look for powdered barley grass that has been dried at a low temperature to save vital enzymes, vitamins, and minerals, and then mix it with juice or add it to a healthy smoothie.

Basil: A part of the mint family, basil's name is Greek in origin and means "royalty." Basil contains significant amounts of antioxidants and has antibacterial and antimicrobial properties. It has been shown to be particularly good at killing harmful bacteria on produce. Throw a few basil leaves in your salad to boost flavor and food safety. Basil helps people adapt to stress by boosting immunity and the body's reaction to stress hormones. It has also been proven helpful in preventing heart disease. *See also* **Tulsi.**

Bean Curd; Tofu: Bean curd, or tofu, is made by coagulating soymilk into a thick curd. Tofu is high in protein and iron and is a rich natural source of calcium and magnesium. Some types of tofu may also be enriched with vitamin D, calcium, and magnesium. Because many soy foods are highly processed, fresh or handmade tofu is the most healthful and can be found in Asian specialty markets and health food stores. Packaged tofu's firmness—soft, firm, or extra firm—depends on the degrees of pressing and water removal. Before refrigeration, tofu is often fermented to keep it from spoiling. Fermented bean curd is very pungent and also contains beneficial bacteria. *See also* **Tempeh** and **Natto.**

Beans, Green: *See* **Green Bean.**

Bee Pollen: Bee pollen contains high concentrations of complete protein (about 35 percent); vitamins A, B, C, D, and E; minerals; and twenty-two amino acids. Although little formal research has been conducted on bee pollen, it has many anecdotal healing properties. Some preliminary studies have demonstrated that bee pollen has antioxidant capabilities, may protect against radiation, and can help promote cellular growth and development. Women who are suffering menopausal symptoms may find relief in bee pollen. In double-blind studies, bee pollen has been shown to relieve many symptoms associated with menopause. Bee pollen has also long been used as a natural remedy for symptoms of flower pollen allergies. For best results, use bee pollen acquired in close proximity to where the allergic reaction originates. Take in small, regular doses to build immunity over time. With more than five thousand enzymes and coenzymes, bee pollen has detoxifying properties. For fresh bee pollen, look in the refrigerated section of the health food store. Bee pollen can also be found in raw, unfiltered honey, but this product has a high sugar content.

Beet (root and greens): Sweet-tasting and low in calories, beets are high in minerals like potassium, iron, and calcium. Beets come

ORAC Score

A test tube analysis that measures antioxidant levels of food, ORAC stands for Oxygen Radical Absorbance Capacity. Foods that contain high levels of antioxidants help protect cells from oxidative damage. Natural body functions such as digestion and physical activity can cause oxidative damage through the formation of free radicals. Free radicals act like slam dancers on a dance floor—crashing into other dancers or cells and creating damage until the free radical is stopped by an antioxidant. Exposure to chemicals, pollution, excess sun, even stress creates damaging free radicals as well. Antioxidants in foods help to quell the damage created by free radicals. An ORAC score measures a food's potential ability to protect against oxidative damage. ORAC scores vary widely from chocolate at 28,000 to carrots at 210 per 100 grams.

in several colors and are an especially good source of folate. Be-tacyanin, a powerful cancer-fighting compound, gives beets their bright color. Traditionally beets have been used to stimulate the liver and help it release stored toxins. Raw beets are particularly detoxifying and are known to be effective blood purifiers. Beets contain numerous antioxidants, including luteolin and betanin. Luteolin has been shown in recent studies to possibly reduce the risk of Alzheimer's disease and to protect against ovarian cancer. Betacynin was shown in research to possibly inhibit oxidation of LDL cholesterol. Other studies have shown that consuming beets may slow the growth of skin and lung tumors. Accord-ing to Ayurvedic dietary recommendations, cooked beets have a calming effect. Don't throw away the bitter greens attached to beetroots! Eat them soon after purchasing or picking, as they per-ish much more quickly than the beets themselves. They can help improve blood and liver function, and you'll get lots of vitamin C, calcium, and iron as well as copious amounts of phosphorus when you forage on beet greens.

Bell Pepper: Bell peppers' spectrum of colors and flavors all de-pend on the stage of ripeness when pepper was picked. Green bell peppers are the least ripe of all bell peppers; yellow bell peppers are sweeter and more ripe than green ones; red peppers contain three times as much vitamin C as green ones do, and are the sweetest and ripest of the three. In general, bell peppers are low in calories; high in vitamins C and B6, folate, beta-carotene, and fiber; and one of the top ten antioxidant vegetables with an ORAC score of 710 per 100 grams. Because conventional pep-pers are heavily treated with pesticides, it is advised to grow, purchase, and consume only organic bell peppers. Eating bell peppers reduces the risk of developing cataracts. They also contain flavonoids and capsaicin. *See also* **Chili Pepper** for more information on capsaicin.

Bitter Melon: Bitter melon looks like a cucumber with warts. Most often served cooked, it is actually a fruit with a history of medicinal uses in India, South America, Japan, China, and the Philippines. Amazonian healers and Ayurvedic physicians have been treating diabetes with bitter melon for thousands of years. And with diabetes levels rising to epidemic proportions around the world, ongoing scientific research is focusing on this bitter gourd's ability to stop this degenerative disease. Some studies have already affirmed bitter melon's ability to remedy hypoglycemia. Charantin, a phytochemical in bitter gourds, has been found to be more powerful than some commonly prescribed pharmaceuticals in its ability to lower blood sugar levels. Polypeptide-p, a compound in bitter melon, mimics the effects of insulin and has been recommended as a natural alternative to insulin shots.

Bitter melon juice or tea has been traditionally used to treat diarrhea, wounds, infections, and parasites in the Amazon. The melon contains antiviral proteins, which have been shown to be useful in treating HIV and tumors. There is some evidence of bitter melon's anticancer properties, and further research into this unique fruit may evidence even more cures. ➤➤ *Preparation tip:* Add bitter melon to vegetable or beef stew. Or try bitter melon Bengali style: Sauté bitter melon and serve with rice as a first course—bitter tapas to get the digestive juices flowing. Medical doctor and raw food advocate Gabriel Cousens has had remarkable success treating diabetes with a raw food diet. He recommends drinking this blood sugar stabilizing tonic: juice 2 ounces fresh bitter melon and combine with fresh cucumber, celery, and lemon juices.

Black Bean: A variety of the common bean, these dark beans are extremely low in fat and high in protein, fiber, and complex carbohydrates. Black beans are a favorable food for anyone with high cholesterol or blood sugar issues, as fibrous legumes help lower cholesterol and keep blood sugar from rising too quickly after a meal. Black beans have significant amounts of antioxidants as well as vitamin B6, folate, and magnesium. A four-year survey of nearly one hundred thousand women showed that those who had higher intakes of common beans have a lower incidence of breast cancer. ⇥ *Preparation tip:* Make black beans more digestible by soaking them for at least eight hours, then draining and cooking in fresh water.

Black Currant Oil: A remedy for arthritis and diarrhea in European folk medicine, black currant oil is still recommended today by many naturopathic doctors for arthritis as well as a wide variety of ailments. Gamma-linolenic acid (GLA) and omega-3 oils, which are both found in black currant oil, are broken down by the body to create prostaglandins, hormone messengers that block pain and initiate many other bodily functions. Black currant oil may decrease inflammation, ease symptoms associated with premenstrual syndrome and menopause, and lower blood pressure. As an anti-inflammatory agent, black currant offers relief to those suffering from rheumatoid arthritis.

Blackberry: A vital berry that easily grows wild even in urban environments, blackberries are closely related to raspberries and are members of the rose family. In Chinese medicine, blackberries are classified as blood-building. A little sweeter than other berries, blackberries have slightly less vitamin A and C. Several notable polyphenolic compounds in blackberries, such as ellagic acid, tannins, quercetin, and others, have been known to regenerate liver cells. Blackberries also have folate and minerals such as potassium, zinc, and manganese. A record-breaking ORAC score of a whopping 5,347 per 100 grams makes blackberries one of the most antioxidant-rich fruits per serving, second only to acai berries. Fresh blackberry juice has been used traditionally as a laxative.

Black-Eyed Pea: Popular in Southern cooking, black-eyed peas are rich in calcium, folate, and vitamin A. Look to black-eyed peas to provide healthy fiber, both soluble and insoluble, as well as antioxidants and protein. Black-eyed peas share health benefits with common beans, such as black beans. *See also* **Black Bean.**

Blood Orange: Blood oranges have all the benefits of oranges, plus anthocyanins. The flavonoids that give plants, including fruits and vegetables, their red and purple colors, anthocyanins may prevent cancer, slow aging, stop inflammation, and prevent diabetes and bacterial infections. *See also* **Orange.**

Blueberry: Native Americans and Icelanders have consumed antioxidant-rich blueberries for their healing powers for thousands of years. In modern times, blueberries' health benefits have been well-publicized. Anthocyanin flavonoids in blueberries give them their dark color and provide copious amounts of antioxidants, are good insurance against heart disease, have anti-inflammatory properties, and can help reduce blood pressure levels. Blueberries are also are plentiful in vitamins C and E, fiber, riboflavin, and manganese. Ellagic acid and other phenolic acids in berries have antiviral and antibacterial properties. Animal studies have shown ellagic acid to have anticancer properties.

Blue-Green Algae: Wild blue-green algae, known scientifically as *Aphanizomenon flos-aquae,* is a nonflowering water plant that grows in inland waters around the world and can be eaten as a dried powder, sprinkled on food, stirred into liquids, or mixed into blender drinks. Aztecs, Incas, and Chinese herbalists consumed algae for its bounty of minerals, vitamins, and medicinal properties. Blue-green algae has unique biological characteristics. It performs photosynthesis like plants, yet even more efficiently. It has soft, digestible cell walls just like animals. And like bacteria, blue-green algae cells lack a membrane-bound nucleus. For these reasons, blue-green algae is nutritious and extremely easy to absorb and digest. What looks like pond scum has properties of a superfood. Dr. Gabriel Cousens's favorite brand of blue-green algae is E3Live. Cousens finds that quality blue-green algae is a whole food that feeds the nervous system, brain function, and even quality of consciousness. Steve Gagne, author of *Food Energetics*, would agree: "Algae assists in the unfolding of stuffed, hardened and accumulated experiences," he explains. According to him, blue-green algae is one of the earth's most primitive life forms, so those who eat it will connect to their deepest primal meaning and purpose. Scientific research suggests blue-green algae boosts immunity, has antioxidant, antiviral, antimutagenic, and anti-inflammatory properties. High in chlorophyll, it has been reported anecdotally to help with weight loss, calming, and antiaging. Grown at Klamath Lake, Oregon, E3Live blue-green algae and other algae have special healing qualities because they spring from the volcanic sediment present in the lake. Blue-green algae has a nutritional balance that bolsters the immune system and enhances brain and emotional functions—not bad for green slime.

Borage Oil: Borage seed oil is one of the most potent sources of gamma-linolenic acid (GLA) of any seed oil. Naturally anti-inflammatory, it has traditionally been used to treat arthritis, skin conditions, and respiratory inflammation. Studies have confirmed borage oil's efficacy in treating rheumatoid arthritis. A German study demonstrated that borage oil may help combat dry skin and itching associated with aging. A typical Western diet contains very little GLA. The three richest sources of this omega-6 fatty acid—black currant oil, evening primrose, and borage oil—protect against degenerative diseases, especially those in which inflammation plays a part. Of these three sources, borage oil contains the largest percentage of GLA and contains no omega-3 fatty acids.

Brazil Nut: Brazil nut trees are part of a rain forest ecosystem. Harvesting wild Brazil nuts creates a viable way of living for many people in the Amazon basin, and provides an alternative to deforestation to create grazing land for cattle, logging, and roads. Brazil nuts contain magnesium and thiamine and are the world's richest food source of selenium, which offers unique protective benefits, such as decreasing the risk of many types of cancer, type 2 diabetes, and heart disease. ➤➤ *Preparation tip:* Always buy fresh Brazil nuts and store them in the freezer or refrigerator. Brazil nuts' high fat content will cause them to easily go rancid. Chop nuts into small pieces and sprinkle them on breakfast cereals, pastas, salads, and desserts.

Brewer's Yeast: Brewer's yeast was originally a by-product of beer making. In the Middle Ages, infants were fed the cloudy sediments left over from beer brewing because this seemed to help them stay healthy. Nutritionists now know that the yeast used in beer making contains health-promoting B vitamins. Because they are abundant in animal proteins yet rare in other foods, brewer's yeast is an important vegetarian source of vitamin B and all elements of vitamin B complex, pantothenic acid, thiamine and riboflavin, niacin, folate, and protein. It has been shown to lower triglyceride levels and raise beneficial HDL cholesterol while lowering detrimental LDL cholesterol. Studies have shown consuming brewer's yeast helps to alleviate symptoms of acne—most likely due to its high chromium content. Brewer's yeast has also been shown to help regulate blood sugar levels, but it has high levels of purine, making it an unadvisable food for anyone suffering from gout, kidney disease, or arthritis. Diabetics should consult with a knowledgeable doctor or health practitioner before using chromium-enriched brewer's yeast, as the combination of niacin and chromium has a notable effect on blood glucose and insulin levels. It is available in powder, flake, bud, or pill form. ➤➤ *Preparation tip*: Add brewer's yeast to soups and tomato-based sauces or smoothies. Brewer's yeast is delicious on popcorn.

Broccoli: A cruciferous vegetable praised for its remarkable anticancer properties, broccoli is high in antioxidants, beta-carotene, and vitamins C and E. Also an exceptionally good source of iron and folic acid, broccoli is rich in minerals such as calcium and zinc. Related to broccoli and sharing similar health benefits are broccolini, broccoli rabe, and broccoli sprouts. Broccoli is also a rich source of lutein, which has anticancer properties of its own. Age-related macular degeneration can be prevented by eating plenty of vegetables like broccoli that contain both zeaxanthin and lutein. Compounds in broccoli called glucosinolates may decrease the excretion of 2-hydroxyestrone, the estrogen linked to breast cancer. Preliminary research shows that one must eat 2 pounds of broccoli per week to cut the risk of cancer in half. However, broccoli sprouts have been found to contain anywhere from thirty to fifty times the protective compounds in mature broccoli plants and are therefore eaten therapeutically by informed people who wish to reduce their risk for cancer. ➤➤ *Preparation tip:* Steam or sauté broccoli, Broccolini, or broccoli rabe. Serve sprouts with salads. Puree broccoli with vegetable broth and ghee for a delicious soup.

Brown Rice: Organic unpolished brown rice is a good source of thiamine, manganese, magnesium, niacin, phosphorus, potassium, iron, selenium, and riboflavin. Plentiful in many beneficial plant compounds, including lignans and phytoestrogens, brown rice is the least allergenic grain. The outer layer of the bran, germ, and endosperm contains fiber and nutrients not found in white rice. An important antioxidant found in brown rice, gamma-oryzanol, has been used as an extract to treat high cholesterol, menopausal symptoms, and digestive disorders.

Brussels Sprouts: A member of the important Brassica genus, brussels sprouts are tiny cabbages that share the same healing properties as other cruciferous vegetables. Low in calories and high in fiber, brussels sprouts' ORAC score is 980 per 100 grams, impressive for a vegetable. Like other cruciferous vegetables, brussels sprouts are rich in vitamin C and antioxidants. Consume brussels sprouts and broccoli to prevent many forms of cancer, especially prostate and breast cancer. *See also* **Cabbage.**

Buckwheat: Not commonly eaten in the United States, buckwheat is a staple food in Russia and Brittany. An extremely hardy plant, buckwheat can be grown easily without excessive pesticides; it will not survive when sprayed with chemicals. Sweet in flavor, buckwheat is actually the seed of the buckwheat fruit and not a cereal grain. An abundant source of rutin, buckwheat strengthens capillaries and blood vessels, reduces blood pressure, and increases circulation to the hands and feet. Another important and powerful flavonoid found in buckwheat is quercetin, also found in apples and onions. A very good source of magnesium, buckwheat also contains protein, phosphorus, manganese, and fiber. Diets that include buckwheat have been associated with lower levels of unhealthy cholesterol and blood pressure. Roasted buckwheat groats are known as kasha and are one of the few alkalizing grains. Sprouting buckwheat multiplies its nutritional content exponentially. Fresh buckwheat greens are also rare in most American markets, but are an excellent source of chlorophyll, enzymes, and vitamins. ➤➤ *Preparation tip:* Make buckwheat breakfast cereal.

Buckwheat Flour: A gluten-free flour, buckwheat flour is used in buckwheat pancakes and, when unprocessed, has the same nutritional content as buckwheat.

Burdock Root: A venerated root in many Asian cuisines, especially Japanese, Korean, Hawaiian, and macrobiotic diets, this dark, woody root that belies its similarity to a witch's finger has many healing properties. Burdock root contains polyacetylenes, phytochemicals that are antibacterial and antifungal. Burdock root contains hyaluronic acid, which supports joint and eye health. Traditional Chinese medicine and Ayurveda use burdock to treat congestion and fever caused by cold or flu. According to Ayurvedic medicine, burdock acts as a blood cleanser.

An excellent detoxifier, burdock root may break up fatty deposits that result in arteriosclerosis. Burdock helps eliminate toxins from the blood, liver, kidneys, lymphatic system, and gallbladder. One study indicated that animals who consumed burdock were protected from the effects of poisonous chemicals. Burdock root is now being studied as a treatment for cancer. The prophetic eleventh-century theologian and healer Hildegard of Bingen used burdock to treat tumors. One recent study demonstrated that arctigenin, a compound in burdock, slows tumor growth. ⇥ *Preparation tip:* Steam burdock root and serve mashed with olive oil, ghee, or butter. Sauté burdock root in stir-fry. Raw burdock root is very pungent, but it can be added to a vegetable juice mix to make an excellent detox drink.

Butterhead Lettuce: Butterhead lettuce is a great salad green that pairs well with more bitter greens. Like most lettuces, it contains water, chlorophyll, folate, vitamins K, A, and C. Lettuces like butterhead are a good raw food addition to any diet and will help offset acid-forming foods like meat, dairy, and other proteins.

Buttermilk: Because it promotes healthy bacteria in the gut, Ayurvedic practitioners recommend buttermilk to alleviate indigestion and constipation. Once a popular health drink in the southern United States, buttermilk has the same gastrointestinal benefits as yogurt. Soured milk, or buttermilk, is fermented cow's milk, so certified organic buttermilk produced from grass-fed cows that do not consume growth hormones is best.

Cabbage: Long studied for its anticancer properties, cabbage usually comes in three different colors: green, red, and purple. A great source of the powerful glucosinolates known to fight cancer, cabbage is recommended by the American Cancer Society for reducing the risk of cancer, along with other cruciferous vegetables such as broccoli, brussels sprouts, and cauliflower. Cruciferous veggies contain goitrogens, which in some cases can interfere with thyroid function, especially when iodine levels in the body are low, so if you are consuming great quantities of cruciferous vegetables, it is advisable to make sure you're getting enough iodine—seafood and all seaweeds are rich in iodine. Green cabbage, especially raw, contains high levels of folate. Cabbage also contains vitamin C, potassium, vitamin B6, biotin, calcium, magnesium, and manganese. Most important, cabbage's rich store of phytochemicals, particularly glucosinates, may be responsible for population surveys which show that cabbage-eaters have reduced rates of cancer, especially of the stomach, colon, lung, and skin. Cabbage also contains indoles, which may help convert estradiol—an estrogen-like hormone that many believe causes breast cancer—into a noncancerous form of estrogen. Sauerkraut and kimchi—essentially fermented cabbage—have their own healing properties, as fermentation creates a probiotic food. Cabbage has been shown to be helpful in the treatment of peptic ulcers when consumed freshly juiced. And last but not least, cabbage has the least amount of calories and fat of any vegetable—making it an excellent weight-loss food. ➻ *Preparation tip:* Shred or cut cabbage into small strips just before cooking, as slicing ahead of time will destroy potent enzymes. Shred a little fresh cabbage in your dinner salad.

Cacao Nibs, Powder: Cacao are pieces of the de-shelled cacao beans. They are bitter and crunchy, and when melted into a paste, used to make chocolate. Cacao beans are often roasted at high temperatures before becoming cacao nibs, but can be produced without roasting, potentially preserving the potent compounds found in raw cacao. Raw or low heat-processed nibs contain the most that chocolate has to offer in antioxidants, flavonols, polyphenols, and phenolics. Cacao nibs and raw cacao powder are high in magnesium and have the highest ORAC score of any food, 28,000 per 100 grams. Look for raw, unprocessed, and unsweetened cacao powder. You can always add your own sweetener. *See also* **Chocolate.**

Cactus Pear: Recent studies in Italy show that the colorful, egg-shaped fruits of the prickly pear cactus greatly reduce levels of oxidative stress in the body, which is one of the main causes of aging. A similar dose of vitamin C was not nearly as effective. Scientists also discovered that the bright and thorny fruits increased vitamin E absorption. Dr. Andrew Weil recommends the psychedelic-colored prickly pear cactus fruit extract to help control blood sugar. ⇝ *Preparation tip:* Fresh cactus pears are hard to find if you don't live in the southwestern United States. Purchase sugar-free jelly made with red, flavonol-loaded cactus pears online.

Cantaloupe: A member of the melon family, cantaloupe is one of the most easily digested foods. Hydrating and cleansing, cantaloupe can replace drinking water for hydration. It's low in calories, and high in minerals like zinc and potassium. Cantaloupe has more heart-healthy potassium than bananas. The zinc in cantaloupe also benefits prostate health. Researchers have found that cantaloupe may have an anticlotting effect on the blood.

Carob Chips and Powder: Health-conscious consumers have been substituting carob for processed chocolate since the 1970s, but carob has been cultivated in the Middle East for the past four thousand years. St. John the Apostle was known for surviving on little more than carob pods for periods of time. Carob lacks theobromine, the stimulant present in chocolate. For those sensitive to stimulants, carob may offer an alternative to chocolate

Food Combining

Simplify the food combinations that you eat in one meal in order to digest what you eat more quickly and easily. Eating a variety of foods in one sitting can be taxing to the digestive system. The easiest foods to digest are melons. Second are all other fruits, then vegetables, and then starches and proteins. Eat the following combinations of foods for better digestion. Food combining is highly recommended if you suffer from acid reflux or other gastrointestinal issues.

> Eat melons alone or with other fruits.
> Eat fruit alone.
> Eat vegetables alone or with starches or
> healthy fats.
> Eat vegetables with proteins or healthy fats.
> Do not eat proteins with starches. (Proteins and
> starches require different enzymes for digestion.)

When you follow these rules in general, you will digest your food with ease, and food will spend less time moving through the gastrointestinal tract.

with a similar, but blander, flavor. In its pure form, carob comes from seeds and pods of the carob plant. It has a unique fiber content that's rich in pectin, lignans, and polyphenols. Caromax, a fiber product made from carob, may reduce unhealthy cholesterol levels. Tannins present in carob have an astringent effect on the gastrointestinal tract and may explain why many alternative practitioners recommend carob as an effective treatment for diarrhea. The tannins in carob as well as its unusually large sugar molecules may also explain why people suffering from acid reflux claim relief when carob is a part of their diet. ➻ *Preparation tip:* Look for raw, ground carob powder, chips, or pods. Mix applesauce with carob powder to treat diarrhea in infants and children. Substitute carob chips for chocolate chips in your recipes, but note that some carob chips are more processed than other forms of carob and most have added sweetener and/or powdered milk as an ingredient.

Carrot: Bugs Bunny and ancient Romans loved these sweet orange roots rich in beta-carotene and high-scoring vegetable on the ORAC scale at 210. Carrots' sweet flavor makes them popular with the children who haven't acquired a taste for vegetables with more challenging flavors. With plenty of fiber, carrots are often enjoyed raw as crunchy sticks or grated in salads or other dishes. Carrots support liver health and actually become healthier when you cook them; the heat breaks down the tough cellular walls and releases beta-carotene. Scientifically speaking, eating one serving of carrots a day has been correlated to reduced risk of heart attacks and some types of cancers. The high level of beta-carotene in carrots protects against macular degeneration and the development of cataracts. Beta-carotene consumption has also been linked to reduced asthma incidences brought on by exposure to secondhand smoke. Carrots' high vitamin A content can help protect against respiratory disease and diarrhea.

Cashew: Lower in fat and higher in protein than most nuts, cashews have a slightly sweet flavor. Plentiful in oleic acid, a monounsaturated fat that has protective effects against heart disease and cancer, cashews also contain many minerals including copper, magnesium, potassium, iron, and zinc. People with kidney or gallbladder problems should be aware that cashews contain oxalates and may need to avoid eating these nuts. Cashews are a good source of biotin and the amino acid tryptophan, the primary building block of serotonin—the feel-good neurotransmitter. They are often heated to remove their poisonous shells, but truly raw, unheated cashews are prized for their intact fatty acids and healing powers. Raw foodists esteem handpicked and polished cashews. Elevate serotonin levels with a tasty bowl of cashews.

Cauliflower: Mark Twain called the cruciferous cauliflower "nothing but cabbage with a college education." Chock-full of stress-relieving B vitamins, it is one of the best vegetarian sources of B5, or pantothenic acid. Cauliflower maintains its status as a healing vegetable by providing plenty of fiber, vitamin C, folate, and biotin, and it also contains sulforaphane, a phytochemical that helps the liver produce anticarcinogenic enzymes. Researchers have shown that cauliflower may decrease the risk of rheumatoid arthritis. Look for cauliflower in purple, yellow, or green as well as white and reap the benefits of this wise vegetable.

Cayenne: Typically a red berry that can range in color from purple to orange, cayenne is the more fiery version of mild, sweet paprika. Folk remedies using cayenne date way back and include healing flu, fevers, respiratory and skin infections as well as ulcers. Cayenne has a copious amount of vitamin C and carotene. Capsaicin heats up cayenne and has many documented medicinal properties including the ability to reduce pain and aid digestion. Hot capsaicin stimulates effective circulation, making it an excellent food and spice for heart health. Cayenne also has fibrinolytic activity, which prevents blood clots from forming. Ironically, capsaicin lowers body temperature, which may explain its popularity in tropical regions. Cayenne helps burn off toxins and break up phlegm during a bout of cold or flu. Good news for dieters—cayenne helps increase metabolism and burn off fat! Unlike other spicy foods, which typically exacerbate ulcers, cayenne seems to alleviate symptoms associated with peptic and duodenal ulcers, particularly when paired with turmeric. Capsaicin's ability to reduce pain may explain why cayenne mysteriously makes ulcers feel better. Cayenne also kills bacteria associated with ulcers and stimulates growth of the cells that line the stomach and intestinal walls.

Celery: Visualize the leafy crown worn by Roman dignitaries—it was made of celery. Esteemed by Greeks and Romans, celery is low in calories and high in vitamin C and fiber. An excellent source of natural electrolytes in the form of sodium and potassium, celery makes a good workout recovery food or, if juiced, a sports drink. Celery and celery seed are excellent sources of coumarins, flavonoid compounds that potentially inhibit various forms of cancer and enhance the abilities of white blood cells. Coumarins also boost vascular health by helping to lower blood pressure and to tone veins. Celery may help prevent or assist in alleviating symptoms of migraines because it decreases vasodilatation that occurs with migraines. Studies have indicated celery to be effective in the prevention of various forms of cancer, assisting in healing liver and kidney diseases, gout, and rheumatoid arthritis. Joint pain associated with arthritis and decreased mobility may be positively affected by celery consumption. Luteolin in celery can reduce inflammation that leads to Alzheimer's. Try a glass of fresh-pressed celery and carrot juice for a soothing bedtime drink—celery's a natural tranquilizer good for insomniacs.

Celery juice is also an excellent natural diet drink. Don't forget to juice the leaves, which are more nutritious than the stalk, containing more calcium, iron, potassium, beta-carotene, and vitamin C.

Chayote: Named by the Aztecs, this light green gourd tastes like a cross between a green apple and a cucumber with only one large edible seed. The fruit and the seed of chayote are replete with vitamin C and amino acids. The leaves and root have medicinal value as a diuretic and in supporting the cardiovascular system. Chayote has anti-inflammatory properties, making it invaluable in treating many of degenerative diseases. ➤➤ *Preparation tip:* Prepare stuffed chayote as you would stuffed squash. Julienne strips of chayote, carrot, and jicama to make a coleslaw salad.

Cheese: Cheese contains high-quality protein, calcium, and other nutrients such as vitamins A and B12, riboflavin, zinc, and phosphorus. However, the type of cheese, ingredients, and production method affect the quality and health benefits of all cheeses. For example, organic cheese, made with organic milk, is preferable to cheese produced with milk from cows that have been given antibiotics and growth hormones. What the cows, goats, or sheep were fed affects the cheese as well—some cows are fed corn or other grains, while and others graze on grass. Cheeses made from animals that feed on grass rather than grain are thought to be more healthy because of their fat content. Dairy allergies are common, and some speculate that this may be compounded by modern pasteurization and processing techniques as well as the fact that dairy-producing animals are not typically grass-fed.

Raw cheeses have more minerals and enzymes than pasteurized cheeses, making them potentially easier to digest. Unpasteurized milk contains the enzyme phosphotase, which promotes lactose digestion and makes the calcium in raw milk and cheese easier to absorb. Advocates of traditionally processed and produced foods, like those who follow the Weston Price protocol, consume only raw dairy produced by grass-fed livestock. Many believe that the healthful substances in raw cheese may help combat allergies and boost immunity. Goat cheese is easier for most people to digest, as it is more similar to human milk than cow's milk is. Sheep milk cheese is another healthy choice.

Cherimoya: An unusual heart-shaped tropical fruit covered with green scaly skin, cherimoya tastes like a combination of pineapple, banana, and honey. Avoiding cherimoya's large dark seeds, scoop out the custard-like white flesh to find a fiber-rich fruit containing ample amounts of niacin and vitamin C. Mark Twain called this fruit "the most delicious fruit known to men."

Cherry: In spring Bing cherries turn a deep mahogany red, boosting the flavonoid content that gives them their bright color. The darker the cherry, the more anthocynanidins and proanthocyanidins are present. These flavonoids affect the body in a similar manner to COX-inhibiting drugs such as Vioxx and Celebrex, reducing pain and inflammation. Some studies have shown that eating twenty cherries is comparable to a dose of ibuprofen for reducing inflammation and pain. Ripe, red Bing cherries are sweet and have more calories than sour cherry varieties. Sour cherries contain vitamins A and C, copper, and manganese, and sweet cherries have the same nutrition, with a little less vitamin A. Montmorency tart cherries are a good food source of melatonin, the hormone that regulates sleep. If you want to eat more cancer-fighting foods, cherries should be a regular part of your diet. Tart cherries contain a substance called perillyl alcohol (POH) that seems to be very effective in reducing the incidence of all types of cancer by depriving cancer cells of the protein they need to grow. If you suffer from gout, cherries can help prevent or alleviate symptoms of attacks. Eating cherries or drinking cherry juice inhibits the activity of xanthine oxidase, the enzyme that helps to produce uric acid, which accumulates in the joints and causes gout.

Fresh organic cherries can be quite expensive, but with all that's known about cherries, think of this money as an investment in good health. Try to avoid nonorganic cherries, as they are typically high in pesticide residue. ➤➤ *Preparation tip:* Cherry season is brief. When fresh cherries aren't in season, drink unsweetened cherry juice, mixing it with sweet fruit juices or sparkling water.

Chestnut: Native Americans and early colonists enjoyed this sweet, chewy, high-carb nut. Low in fat, chestnuts are the only nuts that contain vitamin C. A superb source of vitamins B1, B2, B6, folic acid, manganese, molybdenum, copper, and magnesium, chestnuts symbolize both success and hard times to the Japanese. Chestnuts are a good workout food, providing a tonic for muscles, nerves, and veins. As an antiseptic and tummy soother, chestnuts have anti-inflammatory properties. They have been used traditionally to treat fever, convulsive coughs, and other irritations of the respiratory system. As a Bach Flower Remedy, chestnut relieves hopelessness and extreme mental anguish. Ground chestnuts make nutritious flour, and fresh chestnuts are a classic and nourishing addition to Thanksgiving stuffing.

Chia Seed: The same seeds that make Chia Pets grow are actually very healthy! Used as an endurance food by Aztec warriors, chia seeds are mild in flavor and contain plenty of protein. What's really unique about chia is that when the seeds are soaked, they absorb up to ten times their volume in water, forming a gel. This mucilagenous gel helps to slow the rate of glucose absorption, making chia an excellent food for people with blood sugar issues. Chia seeds are rich in alpha-linolenic acid, a healthy omega-3 fatty acid. Dr. Mehmet Oz praises the health benefits of these

What Exactly Is Fiber?

Plants use fiber to store water. Some fibers are structural containers for water and others are water-absorbing or soluble fibers. When humans and animals consume fruits, vegetables, legumes, grains, nuts, and seeds, we are consuming varying amounts of soluble and insoluble fiber. These two types of fiber move through our intestinal tract, helping to clear out debris. Soluble fiber works like a sponge in the colon, soaking up debris and toxins. Insoluble fiber works like a broom, sweeping accumulated waste out of the digestive system. Processed foods, animal proteins, and complex carbohydrates don't move as easily through the digestive tract and can slow down the natural movement of undigested material through the colon. Plant-based fiber supports healthy digestion by helping the gut clear out toxins and expedite the movement of food through the digestive tract.

unique seeds, baking them into tasty chia seed muffins on the *Oprah* show. ➻ *Preparation tip:* Chia seeds are pretty flavorless, so you can grind them up and sprinkle them on food or bake them into muffins or other foods without changing the flavor too much. Add chia seeds—whole or ground—to add fiber, to keep blood sugar levels steady, or to lose weight!

Chicory; Curly Endive: A bitter green with curly leaves, chicory contains heart-healthy minerals magnesium, potassium, and calcium. Chicory contains substantial amounts of vitamin C as well as vitamin A and iron. It aids optimum liver function, supports blood health, and has been used to eliminate parasites from the digestive system. Include leafy greens like chicory in your diet if you suffer from high blood pressure.

Chili Pepper: Fresh chili peppers are loaded with vitamin C, more than 100 percent of the USRDA. The vitamin C content of chili peppers and their ability to break up mucus in the body make them an ideal food to be consumed during bouts of colds, flu, bronchitis, or sinus infections. They contain copious amounts of bioflavonoids and beta-carotene, making them useful for cancer prevention as well as for boosting suppressed immunity during treatment for cancer. Studies indicate compounds in chili peppers act in ways that support the heart and arteries and, when eaten regularly, prevent heart disease. Some research has shown that capsaicin, the agent in chili peppers that makes them spicy, may act as an anticoagulant, preventing strokes as well as blood clots that could lead to heart attacks. Raw chili peppers support circulation, but take precaution when handling raw peppers, as the oil can get on hair and skin when cutting. To avoid irritation, wear gloves and do not touch your eyes or other sensitive areas.

Chocolate: According to Mayan legend, chocolate was created by the god of lightning, who ceremoniously sent a cacao tree to earth with a thunderous bolt of electricity. Throughout history, chocolate has been recognized as a uniquely pleasurable, sacred, and healing food among many cultures. Like the Mayans, Aztecs drank their chocolate as a bitter beverage and believed cocoa was nourishing, uplifting, and a natural aphrodisiac. Today even astronauts with limited rations are allowed to take a chocolate bar into outer space.

All chocolate originates from raw whole cacao beans—the world's most powerful antioxidant food. How these tropical beans are processed is the key to retaining chocolate's powerful healing effects. First cacao beans are picked, then dried and slightly fermented. Next, they're processed into crunchy cacao pieces called nibs, which are made into chocolate "liquor," which is not an alcohol but a liquid chocolate that is solidified and/or ground. Often the beans used to make cacao nibs are roasted, potentially destroying some of the potency of "raw chocolate." The cacao nibs, raw or roasted, are then mixed with cocoa butter (fat derived from the cacao bean) and sugar to make dark chocolate. Milk chocolate is made by adding milk, sweetener, and less chocolate liquor than used for dark chocolate. Made for use in baking and hot chocolate mixes, Dutch process chocolate is treated with an alkalizing agent to neutralize the acidity of the cocoa. Also called European style, Dutch process chocolate dissolves more easily in water or milk for ease in baking, but the process unfortunately destroys nearly all of cacao's antioxidant power. White chocolate lacks all of the extremely potent polyphenol antioxidants contained in other chocolates because it is simply a blend of cocoa butter (fat derived from the cacao bean) and sweetener.

Besides having miraculous antioxidant capabilities, cacao is extremely rich in magnesium, a mineral known to relax the muscles and nervous system and thereby benefit the heart and the circulatory system. Cacao also contains calcium, iron, zinc, copper, potassium, and manganese. Cacao beans contain vitamins C and A, as well as tremendous quantities of phenolic phytochemicals, dubbed feel-good phenols. One such compound found in chocolate is theobromine, a stimulant whose effects may be confused with the effects of caffeine. Contrary to popular belief, chocolate contains very little caffeine.

Chocolate has always been associated with the heart. A growing list of scientific discoveries confirm chocolate's benefits for the cardiovascular system. Dark chocolate and cacao reduce unhealthy LDL cholesterol levels, and people who add chocolate to their diets have demonstrably lower blood pressure than those who don't eat chocolate. Flavonols in dark chocolate have been shown to create a beneficial reaction in the body, such as improved insulin sensitivity and increased blood flow. Chocolate flavonoids help to reduce blood clots that could lead to heart attack or stroke. Saturated fats in chocolate are rich, complex fatty acids that do not elevate unhealthy cholesterol levels. Another important study at Children's Hospital & Research Center in Oakland, California, showed that flavonols in chocolate helped reduce the symptoms of diarrhea, a leading cause of death in the developing world.

Many cacao trees are sprayed with unhealthy chemicals, while rain forests are destroyed to make room for lucrative cacao trees. When you purchase fair-trade organic chocolate, you avoid contributing to rain forest deforestation and unnecessary pesticide use. ➤➤ *Preparation tip:* How the chocolate is processed makes all the difference. Choose your chocolate wisely. Look for bars of dark chocolate with cacao nibs added to get the most benefit from your chocolate. Chocolate bars made with raw or unroasted cacao are some of the most potent antioxidant foods on earth, but be prepared to pay a premium price for raw chocolate. Another healthy choice is organic fair trade bars from British chocolatier Green and Black's or Dagoba bars—these are made with high-quality organic cacao nibs. Raw unsweetened pieces of chocolate or cacao nibs can be sprinkled on sweet, juicy fruits like fresh peaches or on vanilla ice cream or yogurt. Their crunchy texture and bitter chocolate flavor blends well with sweet soft foods and makes an explosively antioxidant snack. *See also* **Cacao Nibs**.

Cinnamon: Did you know that cinnamon is actually bark from a tree native to Sri Lanka? After the bark is peeled off the tree, it curls into quills we call cinnamon sticks. Long known to be a carminative spice that reduces bloating and gas, cinnamon's chief active ingredient is methylhydroxy chalcone polymer. Essential oils uniquely found in cinnamon have also been found responsible for extraordinary and diverse medicinal uses. With worldwide incidence of diabetes reaching epidemic proportions, cinnamon is receiving attention for its powerful ability to control blood sugar. Adding ground cinnamon to your diet may reduce fasting blood sugar levels by up to 25 percent. Other reported uses of cinnamon include treatment for arthritis, asthma, cancer, diabetes, diarrhea, heart problems, insomnia, PMS, and muscle cramps. Research has confirmed many of cinnamon's extensive uses in traditional and folk medicine. Cinnamon has been found to be an effective muscle relaxant, digestive aid, antibiotic, and antiulcer food. Rich in manganese, cinnamon can help control blood pressure. Cinnamon may also give relief from symptoms of colds and flu. ⇢ *Preparation tip:* Grind fresh cinnamon and then keep it on your table or in the front of your spice shelf. Use it daily to help the body process sugar. Susan Smith Jones, author of *The Healing Power of Nature Foods,* recommends adding a cinnamon stick to a water bottle. The water absorbs the delicious flavor as well as the healing properties of cinnamon. Keep the same stick in a container, adding purified water as needed. When the cinnamon stick uncurls, add a new one.

Cloves: The unopened buds of the clove flower, cloves are a warming spice and contain a unique compound called eugenol. Cloves can be used as mild painkillers and to fight bacterial infections. They also help shield the body from environmental toxins and fight inflammation.

Cocoa Butter: Unlike saturated fats derived from animal products, cocoa butter, extracted from the cacao bean, is believed to be a cholesterol-neutral saturated fat. Cocoa butter contains plant sterols sitosterol and stigmasterol, which may even help reduce unhealthy cholesterol. A large percentage of cocoa butter is oleic acid, the heart-healthy fat found in olive oil. Stearic acid also present in cocoa butter has been found to have a neutral effect on cholesterol. As a complex plant-based saturated fat, cocoa butter is the main ingredient in white chocolate and is often used as a body moisturizer. Formerly chocolate was required to contain cocoa butter, but in late 2008, the FDA changed the rules for chocolate. Buyer beware: now Hershey's and other chocolates may be made with less expensive and much less healthy vegetable oil.

Coconut: In the Philippines the coconut palm is called the tree of life. All parts of the tree are used for practical and medicinal purposes, including coconuts, coconut palm leaves, bark, and roots. Mature coconuts are round with a hairy brown shell and contain rich, nutritious meat. Less mature "young coconuts" contain coconut "water" and have sweet, soft, delicious flesh inside. Young coconuts look like a giant white pencil tips. Inside their hard outer shell is a tasty, sweet liquid, dubbed nature's perfect soft drink. The meat of young coconut can be scraped from the inside of the tough outer shell and makes a delicious ingredient in smoothies and raw desserts. Naturally sweet and great for diabetics, coconut water supports the thyroid gland. Drink fresh or canned young coconut water to curb symptoms of diarrhea. Made from the meat of mature coconuts, many recipes call for shredded coconut. Read your labels carefully and avoid sweetened shredded coconut or coconut treated with propylene glycol.

Coconut Butter; Coconut Oil: Coconut butter is a saturated fat with a great history as a medicinal food. Ayurveda has long extolled the virtues of coconut butter and coconut plant foods. Although some people believe that saturated fat is not healthy, coconut butter is not only healthy but possibly one of the most healthy fats on the planet. When raw or relatively unprocessed, it has a multitude of healing powers. Over 50 percent of coconut's saturated fat is lauric acid, a rare fatty acid found in breast milk.

Unlike animal-based saturated fats, raw coconut butter has many medium-chain fatty acids, which can be metabolized quickly and efficiently by the human body. "Coconut butter contains no cholesterol and does not elevate bad (LDL) cholesterol levels," according to Susan Smith Jones, Ph.D. Coconut oil is naturally antibacterial, antiviral, and antifungal. It is advised to take coconut butter if one has parasites.

Coconut Milk: To make coconut milk, grate or shred fresh mature coconut meat in a blender or food processor. Soak in water and then strain through a tea towel or muslin cloth to extract the milk. Delicious fresh coconut milk keeps for only a few days when refrigerated. More easily procured and much more convenient, canned coconut milk lacks some of the flavor and nutrients of homemade milk. Both are used extensively in Thai and Asian curries.

Cod Liver Oil: Cod liver oil has very high levels of vitamins D and A. Food sources of vitamin D are rare, as usually vitamin D is generated by the human body through exposure to sunlight. Vitamin D deficiencies have been found to be quite high in Western countries where sun exposure is considered to be a risk for skin cancer. Low levels of vitamin D have also been implicated in higher incidence of many types of cancer, including skin cancer. Not sure whether to sunbathe? Wear sun protection as needed and take your cod liver oil! Cod liver oil also contains essential fatty acids EPA and DHA. *See also* **Fish Oil**.

Collard Greens: Very high in chlorophyll, these leaves boost the body against disorders of the colon, respiratory system, lymphatic system, and skeletal system. Nutrient-dense collard greens are like liquid vitamins and mineral supplements when juiced. Get the big picture: when you eat collards, you are supporting eye health and vision. Steer clear of collards if you have a history of kidney stones or gout—they have a high oxalate content, and oxalates will interfere with calcium absorption. Collard greens are an excellent vegan calcium source if you boil them for at least 6 minutes to get rid of oxalates.

Colostrum: Typically collected in the first seventy-two hours after a cow gives birth, bovine colostrum is very similar to human colostrum. It contains unique immune-boosting properties known as transfer factors. Because colostrum helps a newborn grow in its first few hours or days, it contains powerful growth factors that greatly increase the body's ability to repair skin, muscle, and cartilage. Bovine colostrum also contains vital nutrients and anti-inflammatory, antiviral, antifungal, and antioxidant compounds. Because colostrum has so many regenerative properties, many take it as an antiaging tonic. Widely used for combating immune-related chronic diseases such as AIDS and cancer, colostrum has immunoglobulins that neutralize toxins and counter microbial attacks. Bovine colostrum can be found in health food stores, fresh or in tablet powder or capsules.

Corn: A good source of fiber, vitamin B1, folate, vitamin C, and pantothenic acid, corn was a valued food in Mayan, Aztec, Incan, and Native American cultures. Corn is the only grain that contains significant amounts of vitamin A. Today yellow corn is most prevalent, yet before this crop was commercially grown, corn came in a multitude of vibrant hues, such as pink, red, black, and blue. Corn was esteemed in North and Central America for its healing properties, long before scientists could determine the number of calories or micronutrients present in corn. Blue corn, indigenous to the southwestern United States and which the Hopi and Navajo used as a staple food, has made a comeback in recent years. Mostly available in the form of processed snack foods, blue corn has 21 percent more protein, 50 percent more iron, and twice as much manganese and potassium as yellow or white corn. Unfortunately, blue corn chips are so processed that much of the blue corn's nutritional value has been lost. Eating corn supports heart health and reduces the risk of colon cancer by providing significant amounts of folate per serving. Corn and other orange-red carotenoid foods have been shown to lower the risk of developing lung cancer. Traditionally, corn was cooked with limestone or pot ash (calcium oxide), a substance that makes niacin or vitamin B3 available to the body when added to corn. Early American settlers ignored traditional preparation of corn, and many found themselves suffering from pellagra, or niacin deficiency, as a result. *Masa harina* is finely ground white corn flour treated with lime and usually used to make tortillas.

Cranberry: Astringent berries with a long history of medicinal uses, cranberries are replete with vitamin C, soluble and insoluble fiber as well as the trace minerals copper and manganese.

Native Americans recognized cranberries' healing properties, ate them as food, made medicines with them, and used them in ceremonies. The indigenous tribes of the eastern seaboard used cranberries as poultices to heal poison arrow wounds and to cure urinary tract infections and other illnesses. Scientific studies have confirmed that cranberries prevent bacteria from adhering to the lining of the bladder, thereby preventing infections. One of three fruits native to North America that are now commercially grown in the United States, cranberries' bright color stems from their high content of anthocyanidins, the antioxidant pigments found in berries. Long before Power Bars were available, Native Americans had a need for a similar food that would sustain hunters on long expeditions and wouldn't easily spoil. East Coast Native Americans dried deer meat and mixed it with cranberry paste to create a nonperishable protein food replete with antioxidants. Because quinic acid in cranberries cannot be metabolized by the body, it helps prevent kidney stones. When the acid is excreted in urine, it increases the acidity of urine and thereby prevents calcium and phosphate ions from forming insoluble stones. A hearty berry that can stay fresh in the fridge for several weeks, cranberries' anthocyanidins have been shown to prevent atherosclerosis, cancer, and other degenerative diseases. Fresh cranberries have a much higher concentration of anthocyanidins than dried cranberries. Cranberries are antiviral and antifungal, and cranberry juice has been shown in studies to inhibit the *H. pylori* bacteria, a pernicious bug that is associated in cases of acid reflux, peptic ulcers, and increased risk of stomach cancer. Cranberries are also low in calories, with only about 46 calories for a cup of whole raw cranberries.

Cremini Mushroom: A flavorful and medicinal fungus. *See also* **Mushroom.**

Cucumber: Cucumbers are high in silica, the substance that strengthens the body's connective tissue. The figurative nuts and bolts of the body—muscles, ligaments, tendons, cartilage, and bone—all need silica for strength. Choose cucumbers of all shapes and sizes for joint health. Mostly made of water, cucumbers are a top pick for juice enthusiasts. They alkalize the body with a nutritional profile high in potassium and magnesium as well as vitamins C and A and folic acid. Resist the temptation to peel a cucumber, even when juicing, as most of the fiber and nutrients are in the skin. Ayurveda considers cucumbers naturally cooling, and their mineral blend may cool high blood pressure. When feeling bloated, reach for a natural diuretic like cucumbers.

Currants: Actually raisins made from small seedless grapes, currants are superb sources of vitamin C, fiber, calcium, iron, potassium, and vitamins A and B. Currants contain ellagic acid, a potent polyphenol that prevents cancer and can reduce unhealthy cholesterol levels. Anthocyanidins in currants have anti-inflammatory and antioxidant properties, possibly even more powerful than those of blueberries. Remember currants as part of a team of berries that help keep cancer away, support heart health, and reduce your chances of getting Alzheimer's.

Daikon Radish: *See* **Radish.**

Dal; Dhal: Dal is an Indian lentil soup or puree that is very easy to digest and assimilate and provides plenty of protein, healing herbs, and carbohydrates. *See also* **Kitchari.**

Date: Looking for more sweetness in your life? Dates are an excellent unprocessed alternative to sugar. With plenty of fiber, B vitamins, and minerals, dates even help reduce poisons and toxins from the body. Dates' cleansing tannins help with daily housecleaning in the body, mopping up the effects of accumulated wastes and exposure to unhealthy substances. Unlike many other sugars or sweet foods, which leave the body more acidic after consumption, dates are alkalizing to the body. For this reason they are a popular whole food sweetener for raw foodists. Dates are rich in the unique polysaccharide fiber beta-D-glucan, which passes through the colon more slowly than any other type of fiber. Dates may help some people lose weight because elimination is slowed and a feeling of fullness is prolonged when dates are consumed. Rich in antioxidants and anticancer compounds, date extract also protects against free radical damage, according to one study, and successfully combats the ravaging effects of a dangerous cancerous chemical, benzo-(a)pyrene. ➤➤ *Preparation tip:* Dates can be pureed into smoothies or cut into small pieces to sweeten cereal or other dishes. One of my favorite treats, Lärabars are raw whole food bars, made with three to five fruits and nuts. They are sweetened with dates, so you'll be getting a vitamin- and fiber-rich, antioxidant, sweet treat when you take a bite.

Dulse: Dulse is a mineral-rich superfood that supplies a salty flavor to food while delivering a windfall of healing minerals, including iron and iodine. Reddish brown, soft, and chewy, dulse can be eaten raw. It also contains plenty of B vitamins, including B6 and B12. ➤➤ *Preparation tip:* Add a few pieces of dulse to a vegetarian sandwich to add a rich, almost meaty flavor. For those fearful of seaweed, dulse comes in flake or powdered form that can be innocently sprinkled on any food that would benefit from a salty flavor. *See also* **Seaweed.**

Durian: A funny fruit that smells like sweaty socks but tastes like a delicious custard, durian has vitamins B, C, and E, and potassium and tryptophan, an essential amino acid. You might have heard of the calming quality of tryptophan that many know is contained in turkey. Because durian is rich in raw fats, raw food-ists are particularly keen on the healing power of this Asian fruit that's banned from bus travel in many cities due to its noxious odor. Plug your nose and enjoy durian's rich sulfur compounds. Durian may lower cholesterol and is known as a blood cleanser. As word spreads about durian's health benefits, you may find it more easily. Look for fresh durian in Asian markets or find durian juice blends in health food stores or online.

Edamame: Often served in Japanese restaurants, edamame comes in pods and can be purchased frozen or precooked in many grocery stores. Fresh-picked soybeans are sometimes available at farmers markets or in specialty stores. Because unprocessed soy or edamame has the highest protein content of any legume, munch on it to get your fill of protein, fiber, nutrients, and phyto-nutrients. ➻ *Preparation tip:* Uncooked frozen or fresh edamame can be boiled in the pod in lightly salted (sea salt is preferable) water until beans are tender. *See also* **Soybeans** and **Bean Curd.**

Eggplant: Truly purple vegetables or fruits are rare, but most eggplants come in this unusual vibrant color. Rich in dietary fiber and vitamins B1 and B6, eggplants are great sources of folic acid, potassium, and other minerals. Purple eggplant skin contains a potent antioxidant called nasunin. Some animal studies indicate nasunin may be particularly protective for the fatty cells of the brain, shielding cell membranes from free radical damage. A blood-building mineral, iron can be safely stored by those that need it, especially menstruating women and children. However men and post-menopausal women can build up a toxic store of excess iron that increases free radical production and has been associated with increased risk of heart disease and cancer. How-ever, nasunin steps in like a garbage collector to bind up and haul away excess iron. Researchers have revealed that phytonutrients in eggplant may work in conjunction with nasunin to lower cholesterol and improve blood flow in the body. ⇥ *Preparation tip:* For a low-fat dish, bake or grill eggplant, as fried eggplant soaks up inordinate amounts of oil and fat. Serve hot or cold in a salad.

Emu Oil: Made from the fat of the emu bird, emu oil is a superb source of the essential fatty acid linoleic acid and contains the omega-9 oil, oleic acid. It seems the emu goes for long periods without eating, so the fatty pads on its back help it to survive these long fasts. The oil derived from the bird's unique energy storage system has powerful anti-inflammatory properties when taken orally. Aboriginal people of Australia have used emu oil topically for thousands of years to treat burns, wounds, bruises, muscle strains, and joint pain. There is also evidence that emu oil is efficacious in treating eczema and may offer relief for those suffering from hemorrhoids. Emu oil makes a great skin softener, especially for very dry, cracked skin.

Endive, Belgian: A delicate vegetable that must be harvested by hand, Belgian endives' typically white and pale green leaves denigrate when exposed to light. A calorie-counter's best friend, each crisp, tangy, and bitter Belgian endive leaf has one—yes one—calorie and is comprised of 95 percent water. Considered a gourmet salad fixing and related to chicory, Belgian endive contains vitamins C and A, calcium, and fiber. Natural healers recommend it for insomnia and to purify the blood. In the late 1900s, a few varieties of rare purple Belgian endive were cultivated by crossing radicchio and Belgian endive. Though difficult to procure, purple endive has powerful antioxidant anthocyanins. ⇥ *Preparation tip:* Substitute bitter Belgian endive leaves for tortilla or potato chips at your next tailgate. Low in calories and carbs, Belgian endive tastes great with dip.

Evening Primrose Oil: Derived from a plant that produces radiant and expressive yellow flowers, evening primrose oil is high in a rare essential fatty acid, gamma-linolenic acid, and is most helpful in the area of hormone balance. Gamma-linolenic acid (GLA) and linolenic acid convert into prostaglandins, lipid compounds so vital to many bodily functions that they are often classified as hormones. GLA's role in creating these hormone messengers helps balance hormones in the body. Evening primrose oil appears to be more efficiently converted into prostaglandins by the human body than any other oil, even those with higher percentages of GLA. Thus, it is recommended to alleviate symptoms of PMS and menopause. GLA found in evening primrose oil has also been shown to have the ability to alleviate symptoms and causes of many degenerative diseases. It helps prevent hardening of the arteries, heart disease, multiple sclerosis, and high blood pressure and promotes liver regeneration. It has anti-inflammatory properties and is used in treating arthritis and other inflammatory conditions.

Fava Beans; Broad Beans: When in season, fresh fava beans are a delicious, labor-intensive treat. They need to be taken out of the pod, boiled or steamed, and finally shelled. These legumes offer a whopping 85 percent of the daily recommended intake of fiber and are a good source of iron and folate. Fava beans' health benefits are similar to the common bean, with a few exceptions. Fava beans contain levodopa, a precursor to dopamine, a neurotransmitter that regulates cognitive and motor functions. Those suffering from Parkinson's disease are unable to manufacture dopamine. Many prescription medications used to treat Parkinson's disease contain levodopa, the same active ingredient that can be found in fava beans. A few research studies have reached mixed conclusions on whether or not fava beans are effective treatment for Parkinson's patients. Different crops of fava beans may contain varying amounts of levodopa, depending on species, growing conditions, and other uncontrollable circumstances. Favas can cause allergic reactions in some people. Those taking monoamine oxidase inhibitor drugs are at risk for blood pressure elevation when consuming great amounts of favas. If you are suffering from Parkinson's disease, check with your doctor before eating fava beans as a part of your treatment.

Fennel: Popular among herbalists and healers, fennel has been used as a healing food since ancient times. A solid source of vitamin C, potassium, and fiber, fennel's licorice-sweet flavor can be tasted in its bulb and feathery leaves. Folate, magnesium, manganese, iron, calcium, and molybdenum can also be found in fennel. Eating fennel or drinking fennel tea can calm digestive upset. Mothers can calm colicy infants by feeding them gripe water, a mixture of herbs and water that includes fennel. And breastfeeding mothers who drink fennel tea may be able to soothe their babies' intestinal spasms by passing phytonutrients through their breast milk. Anethole and other plant compounds called terpenoids contained in fennel are responsible for the vegetable's ability to relieve gas and stomach pain. These same terpenoids also fight cancer and inflammation. Last, but certainly not least, fennel contains phytoestrogens that seem to have a balancing effect on female hormone levels. If estrogen levels are low, fennel will elevate them; if estrogen levels are high, phytoestrogens work to block receptor sites and compete with the estrogen, thereby decreasing its harmful effects.

Fenugreek: Usually considered an herb, fenugreek seeds can also be sprouted and added to soups or salads to enrich the food with medicinal benefits. Used as a traditional treatment for diabetes in Ethiopia and India, fenugreek has been confirmed by scientific research to lower blood glucose levels, making it a helpful seasoning for the many that suffer from dips and spikes in blood sugar

Phytonutrients

Phytonutrients are chemical compounds found in plants. Scientists have found that many of the compounds that help the plants to survive and protect them from disease, infection, and stress can similarly help humans. Sometimes called phytochemicals, phytonutrients are numerous, and new ones are continually being discovered. Many of them work synergistically with other vitamins, minerals, and compounds in plants.

Scientists have now discovered over nine thousand phytonutrients that help plants attract animals, ward off insects, grow in harsh conditions, and harness the power of the sun. Colors in fruits and vegetables help plants attract pollinators. These colors are also phytonutrients that can help humans heal, prevent illness, or even slow down the aging process. Unique fiber that stores water in desert plants like aloe vera can assist diabetics in controlling blood sugar. The same phytochemicals that help the grain amaranth to survive may help those who eat it to survive the harsh conditions of modern urban life.

levels. With an extremely high fiber content of about 55 percent, fenugreek seeds slow the rapid absorption of glucose. Scientists are continuing to examine fenugreek for its role in cardiovascular health. The ability to reduce unhealthy cholesterol levels as well as the risk of heart attacks has already been attributed to fenugreek consumption in some studies. Diosgenin, a phytoestrogenic compound in fenugreek, appears to mimic the hormone estrogen. This compound has potent cancer-fighting properties and may be a hormone replacement therapy for post-menopausal women. In *The Yoga of Herbs,* Dr. Vasant Lad prescribes fenugreek for healthy digestive and liver function. Finally, fenugreek is known as a galactagogue, a traditional remedy to increase milk production in lactating women. ➻ *Preparation tip:* Sprinkle fenugreek sprouts on food daily, especially salads, soups, and savory dishes. Look for fenugreek sprouts or grow your own.

Fig: Long known in the Mediterranean for their healing properties, figs are delicious fresh or as dried storehouses of nutrition. A fruit particularly rich in minerals, including calcium, magnesium, potassium, iron, copper, and manganese, figs are a great source of energy. If you're tired of prunes, dried figs make great laxatives. High levels of potassium in figs can help control blood pressure, and figs are also a particularly alkaline food, steering the body away from an acidic pH level. There is accumulating evidence that certain diseases such as gout, cancer, rheumatoid arthritis, and even osteoporosis may be tied to body pH levels that are overly acidic. Consumption of acid-forming foods such as animal proteins, dairy products, and processed foods must be offset by alkaline foods such as figs.

Fish Oil: The Inuits of Alaska, Icelanders, and Norwegians owe their good health to omega-3 oils in fish. Epidemiological evidence suggests that a diet high in marine fatty acids decreases incidences of cancer and many other degenerative diseases. Salmon, mackerel, menhaden, herring, and sardines are good sources of fish oil because they are fatty fish that live in cold waters. The omega-3 oils contained in the bodies of these fish allow their cells to remain fluid even in arctic waters. The specific omega-3 oils docosahexaenoic acid (DHA) and eicosapentaenoic acid (EPA) can be immediately utilized by the human body, as opposed to plant sources of omega-3 oils, which must go through a physiological conversion process before they can be utilized.

Many experts recommend fish oil as the best source of omega-3 oils because of the trouble some people have in converting plant-based omega-3 oils, such as flaxseed oil. Eating fish has the same benefits as consuming fish oil extracts, but eating great quantities of fish may be cost-prohibitive for some people. Many fatty fishes have a high level of mercury contamination, whereas fish oil processing can extract mercury and other toxins. Consuming fish oil benefits cardiovascular health, decreasing blood viscosity, blood pressure and blood triglyceride levels. Intake of EPA found in fish oil can reduce inflammation and inflammatory disorders such as rheumatoid arthritis. *See also* **Cod Liver Oil**.

Flaxseed: Mahatma Gandhi once said, "Wherever flaxseeds become a regular food item among the people, there will be better health." The emperor Charlemagne even passed a law requiring his subjects to eat their flax! Flaxseeds are also called lin seeds and contain dietary fiber, magnesium, potassium and manganese, phosphorus, iron and copper. The plant lignans in flaxseeds have been shown to have many significant cancer-fighting properties, especially for women. Lignans increase the production of a substance that helps the body release excess estrogen. Flax has also shown promise in the prevention of colon and prostate cancer. Flaxseeds have an extremely tough outer coating, and if not ground properly, they cannot be broken down in the digestive tract. The volatile oil in flax goes rancid quickly, and exposure to air denigrates the delicate omega-3 oils. For these reasons, flaxseeds are best kept refrigerated and then ground immediately before consumption to ensure freshness and maximum nutritional content. ↠ *Preparation tip:* Use a mortar and pestle, food processor, or (specially designated) coffee grinder to grind flaxseeds, and then get creative and start sprinkling the ground seeds on everything from desserts to cereals to salads. Heat and even exposure to air destroys the volatile oils in flax.

Essential Fatty Acids

Fatty acids are the building blocks of all fats and oils, both saturated and unsaturated. There are certain fatty acids that the body is unable to manufacture, known as essential fatty acids or EFAs. Because they must be supplied by the diet, a lack of essential fatty acids can be a major factor in poor health. Conversely, their ingestion can improve conditions such as dry skin, arthritis, and heart disease while also aiding brain health. Essential fatty acids are utilized throughout the body to build healthy, flexible cell walls.

Two types of important EFAs are omega-3 oils and omega-6 oils, which are categorized by their chemical structures. Omega-3 oils have received a great deal of publicity in the last decade as a result of research demonstrating that many health problems and degenerative diseases may be related to a lack of omega-3 oils in our Western diet. Omega-3 oils, by nature, are extremely volatile and do not have a long shelf life.

A commonsense examination of the average American diet reveals that the lack of live food as well as heavy consumption of processed foods make omega-3 oils scarce in our diets. And to complicate matters, plant-based omega-3 oils like flaxseed (alpha-linolenic acid) must be converted into EPA (eicosapentaenoic acid) or DHA (docosahexaenoic acid). Older people have more difficulty with this conversion. Trans fats found in processed foods inhibit the conversion as well. Women of childbearing age are the best at converting plant-based omega-3 oils to EPA and DHA, as the need for these EFAs is very high during pregnancy. Omega-6 oils are found more readily in most American diets, but often are so processed that they are not worthy building blocks for our bodies. Omega-3 oils keep plant and animal cells fluid and lubricated in all climates. Plants that grow in cold climates, such as in Canada and the Pacific Northwest, and coldwater fish from Alaska or Nordic countries, are the best source of omega-3 oils that stay fluid regardless of temperature.

Flaxseed Oil: Flaxseed oil is the earth's richest source of omega-3 oils. A cleansing and regenerative oil, it must be cold-pressed and unrefined, as flaxseed oil is extremely volatile. Flaxseeds contain alpha-linolenic acid—a short-chain omega-3 oil that is converted to the longer-chain omega-3 fatty acids in the human body. Cold-pressed flaxseed oil has the same benefits as flaxseeds but with no fiber and fewer lignans. Because many people are lacking omega-3 EFAs, flaxseeds can be an important dietary addition. A person who is low in omega-3 oils may have stiff or leaky cells, which could lead to a host of related health issues such as allergies and inflammation. Many scientists and health practitioners have theorized that because the consumption of highly processed foods has risen exponentially in the past hundred years, the overall consumption of omega-3s has declined. Consuming flaxseed oil can help those with dry skin and arthritis, while cold-pressed flaxseed oil supports cardiovascular health and helps to keep inflammation at bay. It's also a mood lifter.

Garbanzo Bean; Chickpea: These little sphere-shaped beans are most often eaten in the Middle Eastern dip known as hummus. Garbanzos—dried, fresh, or canned—are protein rich and a good supplier of fiber, folic acid, and manganese. Like many beans, garbanzos get a thumbs-up for fighting cholesterol and improving blood sugar levels. Molybdenum, found in ample supply in garbanzo beans, helps detoxify the body from sulfites, which are commonly used to preserve lunch meats, bacon, and wine. If you are sulfite-sensitive and deficient in molybdenum, you may experience symptoms of anxiety or headaches when you eat sulfite-containing foods.

Garlic: Sanskrit writings record the use of garlic as a healing agent over five thousand years ago. Egyptians, Chinese, and Greeks also used garlic medicinally. A food as well as a popular flavoring agent, garlic acts as a pungent pill to ward off a multitude of illnesses and degenerative diseases, including atherosclerosis, cough, diarrhea, cold, earache, flu, high blood pressure, infection, and toothache. Sulfur compounds in garlic are mainly responsible for its powerful medicine. An excellent source of vitamin B6, manganese, selenium, and vitamin C and a fair source of phosphorus, calcium, potassium, iron, and copper, garlic has antibacterial, antiviral, and antimicrobial properties. And it fights not only bacterial infections but yeast infections as well. Garlic has been shown to help lower blood pressure, keep blood sugar levels steady, and manage blood cholesterol levels. Studies indicate that regular garlic consumption decreases unhealthy cholesterol levels by 10 percent. Those who consume garlic are less likely to get stomach cancer and/or experience hardening of the arteries or atherosclerosis. Raw and lightly cooked garlic contain the most active therapeutic compounds, but they can be challenging to the stomach and hard on those you kiss. ➻ *Preparation tip:*

Mix fresh chopped garlic into salad dressings and dips—their oil content will help to mitigate the pungency.

Ghee; Clarified Butter: Opinions on dairy products are mixed, yet on the subject of ghee, Ayurveda has never wavered. The ancient healing philosophy of India recognizes ghee as a sacred and auspicious food and no less than the very best fat you can eat. While less popular in the West, ghee is recognized in Ayurveda as a substance that helps one return to wholeness. Casein and lactose are removed from ghee during the clarification process, making it suitable for those allergic to dairy or with lactose or casein intolerance. Ghee is slightly alkalizing as opposed to butter, which is acidifying. Anecdotally reported to lower cholesterol, ghee has demonstrated the same effects under scientific investigation in India. Ghee has a high flash-point of four hundred degrees, making it an excellent fat for high-temperature grilling, roasting, and sautéing. It is also used topically to heal burns and rashes as well as simply to moisturize the epidermis.

Ginger: Ayurveda calls ginger a universal healer for its many benefits and because it is believed to be balancing to all constitutions. Traditionally used to treat gastrointestinal problems, ginger aids in digestion of large or poorly combined meals. (*See* **Food Combining sidebar**, p. 30). Recommended for arthritis sufferers, ginger reduces inflammation and rheumatic pain. Powerful compounds found in ginger, called gingerols, may explain its dramatic ability to reduce pain and inflammation. Gingerols also act as natural blood thinners by preventing blood cells and platelets from clotting or clumping. A proven deterrent of unhealthy cholesterol, ginger prevents cholesterol production in the liver. Clinical studies show that consuming lightly cooked or powdered ginger reduces patients' muscular pain and swelling by 75 to 100 percent. Ginger effectively alleviates symptoms of motion sickness and nausea, including pregnancy-related nausea, even the most severe type—hyperemesis gravidarum. Drink ginger tea when you have the flu—it will help break up congestion and mucus in the body. ↦ *Preparation tip*: Store ginger root uncovered in the vegetable drawer of your fridge. Cut a 1-inch chunk of ginger into small pieces, sauté with 1 to 2 tablespoons of sesame or other cooking oil, add 2 cups of your favorite vegetables, and stir-fry or sauté. Add soy sauce to taste.

Goji Berry; Wolfberry: Small, bright red-orange berries that are some of the most nutritionally dense plant foods on the planet, goji berries have become quite celebrated in the last decade in the West. They have long been regarded in the East for their anti-aging, strength-building properties. Harvested by hand, delicate goji berries are also good for sexual potency and great skin. Chinese martial artists have consumed goji berries for centuries to promote superhuman endurance—helping the fruit to truly earn the name superfood. Li Qing Yuen, a man who lived to an extremely advanced age, was purported to have consumed several ounces of goji berries a day. The berries contain eighteen amino acids, all twenty-one trace minerals including zinc, iron, copper, calcium, and phosphorus. The richest source of beta-carotene on earth, goji berries have five hundred times more vitamin C by weight than oranges and are off the charts in antioxidant value, scoring 25,000 on the ORAC scale. As a plentiful source of vitamin B1, B2, B6, and E, the most nutrient-dense and healing goji berries come from the ancient soils of inner Mongolia and Tibet.

Golden Berry; Incan Berry; Gooseberry; Cape Gooseberry:
These robust berries easily adapt to harsh growing environments and seem to pass on this ability to deal with stressful living condi-

tions to those who consume them. More exotic than raisins, their high vitamin and phytonutrient content make golden berries an excellent dried fruit to consume. Packed with antioxidants and large amounts of good-for-you stuff like iron, phosphorus, and vitamins A, C, B1, B2, B6, and B12, golden berries are particularly high in protein for a fruit (about 16 percent).

Incan berries are considered a good source of vitamin P (bioflavonoids) and are rich in pectin. Hundreds of studies on bioflavonoids have demonstrated that they possess antiviral, anticarcinogenic, anti-inflammatory, antihistamine, and antioxidant activities. They make a delicious, tart, and highly nutritious and exotic "raisin." Put some in your pocket for a long hike or add some to a "raw smoothie."

Grapefruit: A citrus high in vitamin C and potassium yet low in calories, one cup of fresh-squeezed grapefruit juice has over 100 percent of the USRDA of vitamin C. Like other citrus fruits, grapefruits' peels are rich in plant compounds called bioflavonoids, important in the prevention of cancer and heart disease. People suffering from rheumatoid arthritis, lupus, and other inflammatory disorders who eat grapefruit daily report that their symptoms decrease. Scientists aren't exactly sure why grapefruit is particularly effective in reducing symptoms occurring with inflammatory conditions, but they believe certain plant compounds in grapefruit block the prostaglandins that can cause inflammation.

Grapes: Delicious grapes come in many color, seedless, and seed-filled varieties. Similar to other berries in their nutritional content, grapes are a strong source of manganese, vitamins B6 and C, thiamine, riboflavin, and potassium. Resveratrol, a phytoalexin that protects grapes from environmental stressors, acts as a potent antioxidant and has anti-inflammatory and anticancer effects. Resveratrol supports cardiovascular health, cleaning arteries by reducing plaque buildup. Want to look and feel younger? Many think resveratrol can help. It has prolonged the life span of mice in laboratory studies. All grapes may not be alike; typically, the darker the skin of the grape, the more flavonoids are present. Grapes with seeds contain other flavonoids that can support vein health, a good reason to eat them. As storehouses of water, whole grapes can quench your thirst when you need hydration. Or drink purple grape juice—potent purple grapes contain healing polyphenols and natural potassium that help control high blood pressure.

Green Bean; String Bean: Green beans are part of the common bean clan, but unlike their bean relatives, you eat the pods. These healthy beans are picked before the inner beans reach maturity, which greatly increases their vitamin C content. They are also plentiful sources of vitamins A and K, folate, and potassium, iron, and manganese. Green beans are good for your bones! One serving provides one quarter of the USRDA of vitamin K, a cofactor in the production of osteocalcin, a protein that has been found to play an important role in bone mineralization. Fight inflammation by eating fresh string beans—their antioxidants, vitamin C, and beta-carotene will do the job. *See also* **Black Bean, Pinto Bean**.

Green Peppers: Luteolin, a flavonoid found in abundance in green peppers, has many healthful benefits. Recent studies showed that luteolin disrupted a key component of the inflammatory response in the brain, suggesting that luteolin in green peppers and other foods has potential for preventing Alzheimer's and multiple sclerosis.

Green Tea: High antioxidant-power green tea is edible! Of course, you can drink tea for the same benefits. Why not try green tea to boost the health benefits of your food and add an exotic flavor? ➤➤ *Preparation tip:* Use green tea in a spice rub for grilled vegetables or chicken.

Green Tea Salad Dressing

1 tablespoon olive oil

2 tablespoons balsamic vinegar

¼ teaspoon ground pepper

pinch of ground green tea

½ teaspoon Dijon mustard

Mix all ingredients and drizzle over salad.

From *The Ultimate Tea Diet,* by Mark "Dr. Tea" Ukra

Guava: High in fiber and containing up to five times as much vitamin C as an orange, this delicious tropical fruit may be hard to find fresh unless you are vacationing in Hawaii. Guavas also have vitamin A and potassium, magnesium, and even some calcium, a mineral rarely found in fruit. Guavas are the best fruit source of the powerful phytonutrient lycopene. Studies show that this antioxidant helps prevent the growth of tumors, especially from lung and breast cancer cells. Researchers have mounting evidence that lycopene can be very helpful in preventing prostate cancer. Guavas have lots of fiber, much more than apples or bananas. They will give those who eat them fresh extra protection from high cholesterol, heart disease, and type 2 diabetes. Become a food detective and seek out fresh guavas in gourmet, Asian, or Hispanic markets. ➤➤ *Preparation tip:* Slice and serve fresh guavas or buy guava juice at your local health food store.

Hazelnut; Filbert: In the Middle Ages, hazelnuts were believed to have mystical powers and were often used to divine the location of valuable minerals. Today, processed hazelnuts are most popularly used to flavor Nutella spread. Hazelnuts have unusually high levels of the mineral copper, a key factor in an antioxidant enzyme, superoxide dismutase, that helps lower cholesterol and protects cell membranes from oxidative damage. Hazelnuts are also a rich source of B vitamins, vitamin E, magnesium, zinc, and iron. When hazelnut oil was added to animal's diets, their cholesterol levels diminished significantly. All nuts are rich in monounsaturated oils and arginine, have been cited in promoting good cardiovascular health, and may help prevent type 2 diabetes.

Hemp: Hemp milk may be the best health food you haven't heard of. Although hemp food products do not contain psychoactive cannabinoid compounds, they are illegal to produce and grow in the United States. As a result, many people do not know about hemp's tremendous health benefits. It is second only to soybeans in plant-based protein content and is one of nature's best sources of both Omega-3 and Omega-6 EFAs. A number of Canadian companies are making hemp milk, hemp seeds, and hemp protein powder. It is an excellent source of omega-3 oils, which are also prevalent in fish and flax oil. Pregnant women and children who need lots of omega-3 oils for brain development benefit from drinking hemp milk. Omega-3 EFAs help lower cholesterol, decrease inflammation, and possibly prevent many types of cancer. Hemp nuts are high in amino acids, omega-3s, and B vitamins. They are also high in protein, chlorophyll, magnesium, potassium, sulfur, phytosterols, beta-carotene, calcium, iron phosphorus, riboflavin, niacin, and thiamine. Hemp protein powder is high in fiber and an excellent source of bioavailable vegan protein. Brimming with EFAs such as omega-3 oils, omega-6 oils,

GLA, ten essential amino acids, vitamin E, calcium, potassium, and iron, hemp protein powder is also a very good source of magnesium, a mineral many people are deficient in. One serving of hemp protein provides almost half the USRDA of magnesium.

Shelled hemp seeds are a complete protein with essential amino acids. Great for bodybuilding vegans, hemp seeds also contain a balance of omega-3 and omega-6 EFAs. Hemp seeds contain B vitamins and minerals magnesium, potassium, calcium, iron, and phosphorus. Raw or toasted, hemp seeds are an excellent source of dietary fiber. ⇢ *Preparation tip:* Add hemp protein powder to your morning smoothie or to your hot breakfast cereal to introduce a healthy, plant-based protein to your diet.

Hijiki: Rich in minerals, hijiki has been named a bearer of health and beauty. While hijiki helps hair and nails grow longer and stronger, its fiber helps cleanse the intestines and clear out toxins. The mucilagenous fiber in hijiki expands in the stomach and intestines, balancing blood sugar and increasing one's sense of fullness, making it a good diet food. Hijiki is a natural diuretic, and niacin and vitamin B2 in hijiki calm the nerves. *See also* **Seaweed.**

Honey: An important healing food in Ayurvedic medicine, honey has been used for thousands of years to help cure everything from cough to insomnia to heart disease. High in antioxidants, honey contains riboflavin and vitamin B6, iron and manganese. Darker honey generally contains more phenolic compounds and therefore more antioxidants. Dark honey's antioxidants make it a good sweetener for those at risk for cardiovascular disease or high cholesterol. How healthy the honey is depends on how it is processed, as well as the health of the flowers the bees use to collect pollen. Flowers untouched by pesticides and other chemicals produce good honey. Don't serve honey to children less than one year old. ↦ *Preparation tip:* To preserve vital enzymes and phytochemicals in honey, don't heat or add honey to hot foods. For best results, purchase raw, unfiltered, organic honey. Nonorganic honey may be less expensive, but may contain antibiotics used on bees as well as pesticides from plants around or near the hives.

Honeydew Melon: Hydrating honeydews have plenty of vitamin C and potassium. They are also a good source of B vitamins and the trace mineral copper. As a supplier of soluble fiber, honeydew melons' fiber acts like a cleanup crew for the colon, removing toxins and excess cholesterol. The combination of a 90 percent water content and potassium in honeydews helps control blood pressure. Honeydews have a natural diuretic ability. ↦ *Preparation tip:* Don't buy presliced melons. Once honeydews are exposed to light, nutrients begin to break down.

Horseradish: A member of the cabbage family, horseradish has been used historically to improve digestion and alleviate pain and symptoms of arthritis. The phytochemical allyl isothiocyanate gives horseradish its pungent flavor and can successfully attack food pathogens like *E. coli.* Preliminary investigation has revealed even more reasons to pass the horseradish—allyl isothiocyanate is also a tremendous antioxidant.

Huckleberry: The huckleberry is like an undiscovered starlet. While blueberries get all the roles as our favorite antioxidant-packed berries, huckleberries may be equaly as healthful—they just haven't grabbed food researchers' attention. But they do have a cult following among foodies and health nuts. Look to the buzz on berries to lead to more extensive study of huckleberries. Slightly more tart than blueberries and with ten crunchy seeds in the middle, huckleberries are well-known in Europe, where they are used to remedy many ailments. They are especially reputed for their role in prevention of diabetic retinopathy. Reportedly, WWII Royal Air Force pilots who consumed huckleberry jam or drinks claimed they had better night vision. You're on to the next big thing when you buy fresh or frozen huckleberries. ⇥ *Preparation tip:* Prep as you would blueberries, but remember huckleberries' flavor is a little more tart.

Irish Moss; Carrageen: Often used to make vegan "jello," carrageen in Irish moss is used as a thickening agent in many commercial foods as well. Like all seaweeds, Irish moss is extremely rich in minerals and contains vitamins A, C, D, E, K, B1, B2, and B12. A rare vegan source of sulfur-based amino acids like taurine, Irish moss is helpful in alleviating symptoms and as a cure for many digestive disorders such as heartburn, indigestion, and peptic and duodenal ulcers. Extremely alkalizing, Irish moss is helpful in the relief and cure of bunions. *See also* **Seaweed.**

Jaggery: Jaggery is an unrefined sugar usually made from sugarcane but sometimes from date palm sap. Sugarcane juice is heated to about 200°F, concentrated, and then molded into shapes that look like upside-down Tupperware. None of the unappetizing and unhealthy chemicals ordinarily used in processing white sugar, such as sulfur dioxide or bleaching agents, are employed. As a result, mineral salts and vitamins are retained in the final product. Jaggery tastes like hardened maple syrup with a little butter and is sometimes eaten alone as a candy. Ayurvedic medicine considers it to be therapeutic for throat and lung infections, and it is used to sweeten and render palatable many other medicinal formulas in Ayurveda. One study concluded that rats exposed to toxic coal and silica dust were protected from lung damage when they ate jaggery. Gandhi gave jaggery two thumbs up—he savored its unique flavor and recommended it as a sugar that released slowly into the body. Jaggery can be used to sweeten dal or as an everyday sugar. Find it online, in select health food stores, or through Indian or Asian grocers.

Jerusalem Artichoke; Sunchoke: A remarkable root vegetable with a flavor and sweet aftertaste similar to that of a globe artichoke, the sunchoke thereby was dubbed an artichoke. Native Americans harvested these tubers, calling them "sun roots." Jerusalem artichokes are plentiful sources of essential minerals such as potassium, iron, copper, molybdenum, and magnesium. Providing an array of B vitamins, Jerusalem artichokes, like globe artichokes, contain inulin, a polysaccharide handled differently by the body than other sugars. Inulin has a sweet flavor but is not metabolized by the body. Instead it provides fiber and healthy bacteria to the intestinal tract by promoting the growth of bifidobacterium, the main live culture in yogurt. Bifidobacterium has its own list of healing qualities and is believed to be most critical in maintaining a healthy balance of flora in the digestive tract. Bifidobacteria inhibit many disease-causing organisms, have demonstrated antitumor activities, and have been shown to assist in lowering serum cholesterol levels. Bifidobacterium supplements are certainly an option, but Jerusalem artichokes provide a whole food source of this healthy bacterium. Jerusalem artichokes taste sweet but don't cause a spike in blood sugar levels, making them an excellent choice for diabetics. Inulin also has impressive immune-enhancing properties, including increasing the body's defense of destructive bacteria and increasing the movement of white blood cells. Jerusalem artichokes can cause flatulence.

Jicama: Joyful and juicy, jicama makes an ideal diet food. Next time you whip up a bowl of guacamole, don't reach for a tortilla chip. Instead, slice open a crunchy jicama root. You'll be getting fiber, antioxidants, vitamin C, potassium, and other minerals.

Low in calories and high in natural water content, jicamas make a great addition to any juice blend. ➻ *Preparation tip:* Try baking or deep-frying jicama—not quite the same flavor as a potato, but lighter and half the carbs.

Kale: We all could use more green food. If you think that speaks to you, then buy some kale on your next trip to the supermarket. Kale can be juiced, cooked, or eaten raw. It is readily available, and it can also be grown relatively easily. A member of the cruciferous family of vegetables, kale is rich in indoles, glucosinolates, and isothiocyanates, as well as the carotenoids lutein and zeaxanthin. As a green food, kale has lots of magical chlorophyll, which oxygenates the blood, improves red blood cell counts, and aids in simple cell circulation and respiration. Kale also is a powerful warehouse of beta-carotene and vitamins C and E, and actually has more calcium than a glass of milk. Additionally, kale's calcium and mineral balance is more readily absorbed in the body than calcium from dairy products is. A true gift of nature, kale is especially recommended for children, pregnant women, and those at risk for osteoporosis. ➻ *Preparation tip:* If you don't like kale, try dino kale chips! Preheat the oven to 325°F. Wash and towel dry (important for crispy texture) one bunch of dinosaur kale. Trim the stems. Brush or lightly spray with cooking oil, a little sea salt, optional garlic salt. Bake until crispy. Break up kale leaves into pieces, or chips. Sprinkle on salads, vegetables, pasta, or eat alone.

Kasha; Toasted Buckwheat: *See* **Buckwheat.**

Kefir: A cultured dairy product that tastes similar to drinkable yogurt, kefir is a fermented, liquid food made from kefir grains originating from the Caucasus region of Russia. It's a superb source of bioavailable vitamins, calcium, probiotic bacteria, and easily digestible protein. It can be made with raw or pasteurized cow, goat, or sheep's milk, which is then flavored or blended with other herbs and spices. Kefir bolsters healthy bacteria in the intestines, making unhealthy bacteria outnumbered. Served regularly in many Russian hospitals, it has been reported to fight many conditions, from allergies to cancer. Japanese research supports kefir's anticancer properties.

Kelp: Pungent and salty, kelp is often recommended as a healthy salt substitute. Its sodium content is mitigated by its abundant supply of iodine and other minerals. Plentiful plant sterols in kelp may be responsible for its cholesterol-lowering abilities, according to Japanese researchers. ⤙ *Preparation tip:* Kelp is mostly sold in powder or flake form. Season foods with kelp or kelp seasoning blends. *See also* **Seaweed.**

Kidney Bean: Sweeter in flavor yet similar to black beans in nutrient profile, kidney beans have diuretic properties and are used in traditional Chinese medicine to treat edema and swelling. These beans are low in fat and high in fiber, protein, and complex carbohydrates. *See also* **Black Bean.**

Kitchari; Khichdi: This heavy soup is traditionally used in Ayurveda for cleansing and healing. Made with a base of mung beans and basmati rice, kitchari balances all people, regardless of body type or dosha. Mildly spiced with a combination of turmeric, ginger, cumin, cardamom, or other flavors, this healing stew is often served during Panchakarma, an Ayurvedic regimen of detoxification and renewal. Panchakarma employs kitchari as a mono-diet to free energy normally utilized by the digestive process so a patient's body can heal and rejuvenate. Kitchari may also be served as a dietary staple during times of illness or eaten as a nutritious main dish anytime. Dr. Jay Apte makes a ready-to-cook kitchari for busy people.

Kiwi: Originally known as the Chinese gooseberry, kiwi was
renamed by the New Zealand government when it launched a
massive public relations campaign to market this fuzzy fruit. Ap-
parently it worked, as the green fleshy fruit is now grown and
eaten all over the world. A significant source of vitamin E, folic
acid, minerals, and fiber in the form of pectin, kiwis also contain
lutein and zeaxanthin—both associated with prevention of macular degeneration. Kiwifruit boosts immunity with 230 percent
of the USRDA of vitamin C. Step aside, bananas! Few people
know that a serving of kiwi delivers 20 percent more potassium
than a serving of the better-known yellow fruit.

Kohlrabi: As a member of the Brassica genus, kohlrabi offers
health protective properties similar to broccoli. In fact, the bulb-
like stem of kohlrabi tastes remarkably like the central stalk of
broccoli, but is a little sweeter and a little less fibrous. Kohlrabi
greens are deliciously edible, but you'll need to eat them quickly,
as they will perish much more quickly than the bulbous stem.

Choose kohlrabi as a way to increase cancer prevention in the form of cruciferous vegetables. Like broccoli, it contains gluco-sinolates, specifically indole-3-carbinol and sulforaphane, which increase the excretion of the form of estrogen linked to breast cancer. ➻ *Preparation tip:* Peel the hard outer skin off the bul-bous stem and slice kohlrabi into thin slices. Serve with your favorite dip.

Kombu: A specific strain of kelp sold in strips or sheets, kombu adds flavor and minerals to soup stock and is often used in Asian cuisine. Kombu contains vitamin A, some B vitamins, and plenty of calcium and iron. Add kombu to your next pot of beans—it will add vitamins and minerals as well as reduce the gas-inducing qualities of the legumes. *See also* **Seaweed.**

Kombucha: Basic kombucha is made by adding a starter culture of yeast, bacteria, acetic acid, and sugar to cooled tea, usually black or green tea. It's then allowed to ferment. The results are a fairly powerful antioxidant and anti-microbial drink that's reported to boost immunity, fight stress, and support the liver. Many producers add flavor and carbonation to make Kombucha an exotic, health-boosting elixir.

Kumquat: Low in fat and high in dietary fiber, the kumquat is a citrus that is eaten whole. Four kumquats provide nearly half of the USRDA for vitamin C. Like all citrus fruits, kumquats have some potassium, helpful in controlling blood pressure levels. Most important, because it's easy to eat the peel, kumquats are an excellent food-based source of phytochemicals called liminoids, which have been shown in studies to stop and even reverse the progression of cancer. Kumquat rinds are so powerful that they reduce the efficacy of the drug tamoxifen and should not be eaten when taking this prescription medication.

Leek: A member of the onion and garlic family, leeks have the same health benefits as their more pungent cousins. Proportionally, you'll need to eat more leeks than garlic or onions to reap the same rewards. Nonetheless, when you add leeks to soups, pastas, and vegetable casseroles, you will be boosting your immune system and fighting cancer. Maybe your breath will be sweeter, too!

Lemon: One of the most ubiquitous and powerful healers, lemons are available at almost every corner store. Why are lemons so great? First, they boost the immune system with a powerful dose of vitamin C. They are so acidic that they rapidly convert to an alkaline pH during the digestive process, making these citrus fruits powerful healers for those who consume an acidic diet. Ayurvedic chef Miriam Hospodar says that lemons stimulate digestive fire and "are both cleansing and nourishing." Lemons also provide vitamin B6, potassium, and folic acid, as well as the powerful phytochemicals limonin and limonene. Found in the pith or white part of the fruit below the yellow peel, researchers have discovered that limonin and limonene have many cancer-fighting abilities. The pith also contains high levels of bioflavonoids that strengthen capillaries. Citrus flavonoids in lemon peels are highly recommended for those suffering from any form of vein collapse, such as varicose veins or spider veins. However, lemon peels contain oxalates, so people suffering from kidney stones or gout should avoid eating lemon zest or peel. Lemons have been shown in studies to be especially helpful in preventing stomach cancer. Potassium in lemons also helps to regulate blood pressure and offset potassium loss from taking blood pressure medication. Drink lemon juice in the morning to purify the liver. ⇥ *Preparation tip:* Boost the healing power of a glass of water by adding lemon juice. Keep slices handy and squeeze them into each glass or bottle. Bioflavonoid Boost: Grate lemon or orange peel, making sure to get down to the white part. Add the zest to a cup of herbal or black tea. Use Meyer lemons and Meyer peels for sweeter zest and juice. *See also* **Lime.**

Lemon Balm: Lemon balm has a long history as a calming and soothing herb. Traditionally used for longevity, lemon balm supports heart health and circulation. ➻ *Preparation tip:* This herb makes a delicious buttery lemon tea, can be served in salads, or used to season seafood and poultry.

Lentil: Because they are small, lentils are one of the easiest legumes to prepare. Their nutritional profile does not stray too far from common beans. Eating lentils will provide you with protein, folic acid, and trace minerals. Probably the most convincing reason to eat lentils is for their health-building fiber. Known to lower cholesterol, lentil fiber also keeps blood sugar levels steady, preventing it from rising too quickly after a meal. Lentils and other common beans also offer the promise of protection from breast cancer. A surprising study conducted in the 1990s revealed that among the 90,630 women surveyed, those who ate beans and lentils were associated with a 24 percent reduced risk of breast cancer. Even more surprising was the fact that other recognized cancer-fighting foods such as tea, onions, apples, string beans, broccoli, green peppers, and blueberries showed no significant protective effect, making eating lentils even more enticing.

Lettuce: So fond of lettuce was Augustus Caesar that he erected a statue in honor of the leaves. Lettuce comes in many textures, flavors, and colors—from iceberg to romaine, butterhead to red leaf. All lettuce contains life-giving chlorophyll and in general, the darker the lettuce, the greater the nutrient density. Iceberg contains choline; romaine has significant amounts of folic acid and vitamins A, B1, B2, and C. Romaine also has minerals such as manganese and chromium. Caesar most likely ate wild lettuce, which was historically known for its calming effect. The milk from wild lettuce leaves contains natural latex that relaxes the nervous system in the same way that opium or poppy seeds work. Unfortunately, modern cultivated lettuce does not have as much of this nerve tonic. A variety of other greens are often added to salads, and many have their own healing properties. *See also* **Arugula** and **Watercress**.

Lima Bean; Butter Bean: Lima beans are very rich in trace minerals manganese and molybdenum, as well as dietary fiber. Hunt for fresh limas in gourmet grocers and farmers markets, or purchase them frozen or, as a last resort, canned. Lima beans are a good source of folate, protein, potassium, iron, copper, phosphorus, magnesium, and thiamine. Eat lima beans to protect yourself from the adverse effects of the food preservative nitrate. Like all common beans, limas help keep unhealthy cholesterol at bay and assist in maintaining steady blood sugar levels.

Lime: Of course green and tangy limes are an excellent source of vitamins C and B6, potassium, and folic acid. But how often do you pass up the potent phytochemicals located in lemon and lime skin? You may change your mind when you hear about limonin and limonene. Present in lemon and lime zest, limonene and limonin have many health benefits. Investigators believe that limonene may activate proteins that help eliminate estradiol, a hormone that has been linked with breast cancer. Other studies show that limonene increases enzymes in the liver that are able to eliminate cancer-causing chemicals in the body. Squeezing lime juice on your food may activate white blood cells and act as an antibiotic. Researchers have also discovered that lime juice is a good guard against cholera, a prevalent health threat in Africa. ➻ *Preparation tip:* When zesting a lime, make sure you use organic limes and only the green part of the skin.

Loquat: Peel a fresh loquat, and every bite will be filled with fiber, loads of vitamins A and B6, potassium, and manganese. The darker the flesh, the more protective carotenoids are present in the fruit. Phytonutrients in loquats may help to prevent macular degeneration. Instead of using cough medicine, try loquat leaf extract, which is used as a traditional cough remedy and tummy tamer in tropical countries. Find fresh loquats at Asian markets or gourmet grocers.

Lotus Root: From the muddy water arises the beautiful and symbolic lotus flower. Below the flower, in the mud, grows the lotus root. Used extensively in Asian cuisine, from soups to tempura, lotus root's unusual beauty adds an artful touch to many dishes. Somewhat resembling the human lungs, the lotus root assists in healing all ailments of the upper respiratory tract, including asthma, bronchitis, and cough. Lotus root is said to melt mucus, especially in the lungs. It nourishes with dietary fiber, vitamins C and B6, thiamine, potassium, phosphorus, copper, and manganese.

Lucuma: An exotic Peruvian fruit from a tree that has been known to reach fertility at the age of five hundred years, raw powdered lucuma can be found in health food stores. Use it as a whole food sweetener that provides flavor and a few bonus vitamins like beta-carotene, vitamin B3, and iron.

Lychee: Known as the king of fruit in South China, lychees are a good source of vitamin C, riboflavin, potassium, and copper. The small, Ping-Pong-shaped lychee, with its strawberry-colored, leathery skin, is often blended into exotic cocktails. Find fresh lychees at Asian markets or gourmet grocers. Use juice or canned lychees when fresh fruit is unavailable.

Maca Root: Before the modern advent of scientifically proven remedies, powerful plant foods like maca were believed by ancient peoples to be magical. Maca looks like a turnip but is shaped like a beet. Used by the ancient shamans of Peru, maca root thrives at an elevation of around fourteen thousand feet, where almost no other plants can survive. Known to enhance the stamina of warriors in battle, maca root can be used by modern athletes instead of steroids for performance enhancement, improving stamina and strength. An excellent source of vegan bioavailable calcium, maca also helps build bones. Maca has a long history of being used to increase libido. A natural adaptogen, maca root is ideally suited to support the endocrine system. Adaptogens either increase or decrease support for hormones in the body. If an endocrine gland is overproducing, adaptogens like maca will help inhibit production of hormones. Conversely, adaptogens help to boost production of glands that are not functioning up to par. Maca root can help balance the adrenal glands, thyroid, thymus, pancreas, pituitary gland, hypothalamus, and ovaries. Menopausal women can often benefit from the hormone-balancing qualities of maca root. Available in powdered form, maca can be added to soups, smoothies, or juice to boost the healing power of these foods.

Macadamia Nut: Native not to Hawaii, but to Australian rain forests, macadamia nut season brought Aborigines gathering ceremoniously to feast gratefully on these delicious, high-fat nuts. Macadamia nuts are a good source of potassium, magnesium, copper, iron, vitamins B1 and B3, lots of vitamin E, and beneficial monounsaturated fats. Like other nuts, macadamias contain arginine, responsible for lowering cholesterol and unhealthy triglyceride levels. ⇥ *Preparation tip:* Many health-conscious cooks recommend cooking with macadamia nut oil because it contains lower amounts of polyunsaturated fats, making it more stable at higher temperatures. In fact, macadamia nut oil is twice as stable as olive oil and four times as stable as canola oil. It may be a little more expensive. Cook foods with a little macadamia nut oil and then add other oils for flavor after cooking.

Mache; Lamb's Lettuce: Mache has been cultivated in France since the seventeenth century. Prior to cultivation, peasants foraged for this low-calorie, nutrient-dense green in the wild. Mache has three times the vitamin C content of regular lettuce, as well as plenty of beta-carotene, vitamins B6 and B9, and omega-3 fatty acids.

Maitake: Mild, brown, fan-shaped mushrooms, maitakes contain protein, selenium, potassium, vitamin C, iron, and fiber. Studies reveal maitake mushrooms may have more tumor-fighting abilities than any other mushroom. In laboratory investigations of mushroom extracts' effectiveness in retarding tumor growth, maitakes came out on top. Beta-D-glucans in maitake mushrooms play a role in boosting immune system response. In test tubes, maitake extract activates armies of white blood cells and increases their ability to destroy cancer cells, microbes, and other foreign cells. Beta-D-glucans in maitakes also stimulate production of white blood cells in bone marrow, critical for cancer patients undergoing chemotherapy or other radiation treatments. Maitake mushrooms and mushroom extract can safely supplement conventional cancer treatment by reducing uncomfortable side effects such as nausea, fatigue, weight loss, and immune suppression. In studies on cancer patients, maitakes have also been shown to prevent healthy cells from turning cancerous and boost patient's immunity. *See also* **Mushroom.**

Mango: Buddha loved this magnificent fruit and often meditated under the branches of a mango tree. Bursting with carotenes, vitamin C, copper, and almost twice the recommended daily allowance of vitamin A, mangoes have one of the largest seeds of any fruit. They are also good sources of vitamin E, potassium, iron, and magnesium. Mangoes are over 80 percent water, and are an excellent source of soluble and insoluble fiber. Sweet and juicy mangoes are powerful storehouses of carotenoids, antioxidants, and phytonutrients. Long before the discovery of chemical compounds in food, Ayurveda considered mangoes the king of fruits. Investigators have found evidence that mangoes may prevent certain types of cancers. In one study on cancer cells in mice, mangoes in a water-soluble solution were 10 times as effective in preventing cancer as isolated mango carotenes. Mangoes symbolize undying love in India, and antioxidant-filled fruit helps the heart and supports a healthy cardiovascular system. Indian healers suggest mango cures anemia, as their high iron content can help build blood. Use mango's calcium and magnesium to prevent muscle cramps. In fact, mangoes are great for pregnant women who need minerals, fiber, water, and antioxidants. ⇢ *Preparation tip:* Mango Lassi: Cut the mango down the middle twice, leaving the seed in the middle. Scoop out the soft mango fruit out of the skin, chop, and put in a blender. Add ½ cup yogurt and 1½ cups water. Blend and serve.

Mangosteen: A tropical fruit with a hard purple-brown outer coating and a soft inner white flesh, the mangosteen is not related to the mango and has very low levels of vitamins and minerals compared to other fruits. What has been fueling a growing market in the West for mangosteen juice and fresh mangosteens is the presence of compounds called xanthones. Mangosteens have over forty different xanthones contained in both the fruit and the hard outer shell. Research on xanthones is still preliminary, but there is evidence that these polyphenols have demonstrated antitumoral, antibiotic, antiviral, anti-inflammatory, and anti-allergenic properties. Before mangosteen juice was sold by multilevel marketers, Southeast Asians used the fruit to cure countless ailments, including infections, dysentery, and skin problems, and to reduce pain. ➤➤ *Preparation tip:* Buy mangosteen juice puree that includes not only the fruit juice, but also the hard outer shell or peri-cap (contains the most xanthones). Buyer beware! Fresh mangosteens grown in Thailand have been irradiated per USDA regulation.

Maple Syrup: First harvested by Native Americans who drove tomahawks into maple trees to extract this rich fluid, maple syrup is used as food and medicine. Native Americans used hot stones to heat maple syrup and thicken it by extracting water. Today, maple syrup is sometimes processed through reverse osmosis filters to remove water and then boiled to reach the desired consistency or grade. Because of its mineral content and minimal processing, maple syrup is considered a fairly healthy sugar. There are three grades of maple syrup: A, B, and C. The lower the grade of syrup, the greater the concentration of minerals. Grade C has the most minerals. A plentiful source of manganese, maple syrup helps cells fight inflammation. Manganese acts as a cofactor in the main antioxidant enzyme of the mitochondria that power up the cells of our body. Also rich in zinc, maple syrup builds immunity, as zinc plays a key role in immune function by supporting the thymus gland. In Stanley Burroughs's *The Master Cleanser,* the recommended healing fast consists of water, cayenne, fresh lemon juice, and maple syrup. ➤➤ *Preparation tip:* Skip the fast and make Master Cleanser lemonade. Pour a glass of 8-12 ounces of water, add the juice of ½ lemon, add ½ to 1 tablespoon of maple syrup and a pinch of cayenne, and enjoy!

Marionberry: This supersized blackberry is really a cross between an olallie berry and Chehalem berry. Grown in Oregon, marionberries are sweet and juicy and have a nutritional breakdown and phytonutrient content closely related to blackberries. *See also* **Blackberry.**

Melon: *See* **Cantaloupe, Honeydew Melon,** and **Watermelon.**

Microgreens: *See* **Sprouts.**

Eat Local

The world has a bounty of healing foods. Sometimes the best eats come close to home. Goji berries harvested from the Himalayas might make you live longer, but so could strawberries grown a few miles from your doorstep. Easier on the pocketbook, local food is not only good for you, it's kinder to the planet. Think of all the energy wasted away by the trucks, trains, and jet planes that travel thousands of miles to bring food to consumers. There is a bounty of healthy foods available from around the world, but eating primarily locally grown, seasonally produced foods has other benefits for your health. The food is usually fresher, and in some ancient healing traditions, the food grown in the environment near where you live has greater balancing and healing effect than food cultivated far away. Look for "locally grown" signs at the supermarket, or shop at farmers markets for the freshest local foods. Even better, grow your own food. Front or backyard and even container gardens can yield a delicious harvest of fresh herbs and produce.

Milk, Cow's: Shunned by vegans and many health food advocates, cow's milk is a revered food in Ayurveda. In the ancient Indian system, cow's milk is considered a building food. While some doctors recommend low-fat, pasteurized milk, members of the Weston A. Price Foundation and others believe unaltered milk is best. In the 1920s, raw milk was commonly consumed in the United States. Advocates of raw milk believe it is less likely to be contaminated by bacteria such as *E. coli* because raw milk is carefully produced on a small scale with safety precautions built in to the system to prevent any contamination. Pasteurization kills many of the enzymes and strains of beneficial bacteria that occur in raw milk. Natural raw milk contains plenty of bone-building calcium, beneficial bacteria, and vital enzymes. Grass-fed livestock may produce healthier milk than grain-fed animals on commercial farms.

Millet: Next time you're craving white rice or baked potatoes, why not try miraculous millet instead? It was the grain of choice in ancient China before rice took over as a favorite. An unrefined grain that is antibacterial and antifungal and aids digestion, there are many reasons to incorporate millet into your diet. For one thing, it has the most complete protein of any grain, and more fiber than rice. Known as the queen of grains, millet is a rich source of thiamine, niacin, and minerals magnesium, phosphorus, zinc, copper, and manganese. Gluten-free millet has been known to soothe morning sickness during pregnancy. In traditional Chinese medicine, millet strengthens the stomach, spleen, and pancreas. Eating millet a few times a week protects against heart disease, diabetes, and cancer. ➤➤ *Preparation tip*: Rinse millet before cooking. Bring 1 cup of millet and 3 cups of water to a boil and reduce to a simmer for 15–20 minutes. Enjoy with stir-fries or vegetables.

Miso: Rich in enzymes and healthy bacteria, miso is a fermented paste made from soybeans, rice, and mold. Fermented foods like miso have benefits for our intestinal flora because they build healthy bacteria cultures in the digestive tract. By varying ingredients and processing techniques, miso has quite a range of textures, flavors, and colors. In fact, miso-making in many Asian countries is akin to making fine wine or cheese. Miso is a good nutritional source of many minerals, including zinc, manganese, phosphorus, iron, and copper. It is a good source of protein and vitamin B12, a vitamin that is difficult for vegetarians to derive from plant sources. Experts are uncertain, however, as to whether the form of B12 in miso is absorbable, and there is tremendous variation in content of B12 in various misos. Teeming with healthy enzymes, lactobacillus, and other microorganisms that aid in the digestion of all foods, miso may be easier to digest than other forms of soy products. Miso's live cultures have been shown to ward off and destroy harmful microorganisms, thereby fostering a healthy digestive system. ➻ *Preparation tip:* Prepare a vegetable stir-fry and serve with ½ teaspoon of miso for a unique salty flavor. Put it on the side or blend it into the stir-fry.

Mung Bean: Recognizable as the most common sprout used in Asian stir-fries, mung beans have a long history of healing. In India, they are often the main ingredient in a medicinal stew called kitchari. Mung beans have been cultivated in China for over seven thousand years and are believed to balance all individual constitutions in Ayurveda. In Chinese medicine, mung beans support the liver and help detoxify the body. Besides being revered in many Asian healing traditions for their therapeutic benefits, mung beans have a similar nutritional profile to that of other common beans. *See also* **Black Bean**, **Pinto Bean**, and **Kitchari**.

Mushroom: Button mushrooms such as white, cremini, and portobello mushrooms share similar health benefits. As fungi, they are all excellent sources of minerals selenium, copper, potassium, and zinc. Button mushrooms also contain some protein, B vitamins, riboflavin, and pantothenic acid. Cremini mushrooms are also good sources of B6 and B12. Phytochemicals in mushrooms have been the subject of much research. Cancer-preventing polysaccharides and beta-glucans can be found even in button mushrooms, but greater quantities of these important compounds are contained in less common mushrooms such as shitake and maitake.

Nama Shoyu: The champagne of soy sauces, raw unpasteurized nama shoyu is filled with vital healing enzymes and amino acids. Often carefully and painstakingly brewed and fermented, nama shoyu shares many of miso's medicinal properties.

Natto: A fermented soybean paste that is said to be an acquired taste, natto is one of the world's most powerful fibrinolytic foods, greatly reducing the possibility of blood clotting. Natto also contains great amounts of vitamin K, helpful in building bone and preventing osteoporosis. It may also be helpful in preventing various types of cancer and lowering cholesterol.

Navy Bean: Named not for their color, but for their role in feeding the U.S. Navy in the twentieth century, these beans were chosen by American naval forces for their high protein, low fat, and nutrient-dense content. Dried beans are easy to store at home or at sea and can cook up into a highly nutritious healing stew or chili. *See also* **Pinto Bean** and **Black Bean.**

Nectarine: *See* **Peach.**

Noni: A tropical fruit that looks like a pineapple turned inside out, the noni, with its thick black juice, has been recommended as a remedy for an endless list of ailments. Wild noni trees grow in such inhospitable places as the cracks of dried lava beds. Noni trees adapt to varied tropical landscapes, and the fruit seems to adapt to heal whatever ails a person. Much of noni's medicinal uses are anecdotally reported or based on information offered by indigenous healers in regions where the fruit grows. Scientific research on noni has demonstrated its possible anticancer effects and confirmed its antioxidant properties. One study showed that mice fed noni experienced increased endurance. Other studies have shown that it may lower cholesterol. Fresh noni is hard to come by unless you live in a tropical region. Many alternative healers recommend noni juice or powder for its nutritive, detoxifying, immuno-building, and endocrine-supporting effects. Noni has been used for such diverse conditions as digestive problems—including diarrhea and parasites—arthritis, inflammation and gout, pain, and cardiovascular issues, including high or low blood pressure or cholesterol. The Sanskrit word for *noni* is *ashyuka*, which means "longevity." ➺ *Preparation tip:* Try high-quality noni powder in your next smoothie.

Nopales Cactus: Filled with soluble fiber, vitamins, and minerals, nopales cactus is one of the best foods a diabetic can eat. Desert plants like aloe and nopales seem uniquely suited to help heal diabetes because the fiber in such plants comes in the form of gum and mucilage. These fibers break down carbohydrates for digestion and help the body regulate blood sugar. Scientists and others aren't sure why, but somehow the fiber and medicinal value of desert plants seems to radically slow or even reverse type 2 diabetes. Most species of cactus also contain large quantities of alkaloids beneficial for alleviating symptoms of diarrhea and other digestive issues.

Nori: Made by shredding and rack drying sea algae in a process similar to making paper, nori is sold in sheets. Used for making sushi, nori contains vitamins C and D, and many B vitamins, including B12. Mineral-rich nori grows near the seashore, making its flavor more mild and palatable than that of other seaweeds. ➻ *Preparation tip:* Cut nori into small pieces and then sprinkle on salads, soups, and sandwiches. Try toasted nori for a delicious treat. *See also* **Seaweed**.

Oats: One of the best sources of silicon, a trace mineral that help renew bones and connective tissues, oats also contain phosphorus, required for brain and nerve formation in children. Rolled oats are quite nutritious, are minimally processed, and are the most popular whole grain consumed in the West. Steel-cut oats, or oat groats, are less processed, take longer to cook than rolled oats, and have a much lower glycemic index. High fiber oats contain more soluble fiber than any other grain, and it comes in the form of beta-glucan—a sticky fiber that mops up cholesterol and sends it out of the intestines. Saponins in oats also work to bind cholesterol and usher it out of the body. They appear to bolster the immune system, too, as a diet high in saponins has been linked to increased levels of killer T cells, the body's first cellular line of defense in battling infections and tumor cells and other cellular invaders. The fiber in oats also helps fight cancer—experts have reviewed more than two hundred studies that linked high intake of dietary fiber with reduced risk of cancer. Phytic acid, a compound in oats that binds reactive minerals, is believed to play an important role in preventing colon cancer.

Okra: Unless you've eaten lots of gumbo, Indian food, or African cuisine, you probably haven't had your fill of okra. Nutrient-rich and low in calories, okra makes for a great diet food. It contains vitamin C, beta-carotene, thiamine, folic acid, riboflavin, calcium, potassium, magnesium, and zinc. A powerhouse of soluble fibers in the form of gums and pectins, okra's gooey, mucilaginous texture soaks up unhealthy cholesterol, toxins, and mucous waste and cleans them out of the intestinal tract. Okra's alkaline slime acts as a laxative, is good for healing ulcers, and may help reduce symptoms of acid reflux. Like all fiber-rich veggies, okra promotes good cardiovascular and gastrointestinal health and helps to regulate blood sugar. Okra contains glutathione, a master antioxidant. Researchers at Emory University found that glutathione in okra attacks cancer by protecting cells from mutation and preventing cancerous chemicals from damaging DNA, clearing these toxins out of the body. Okra, not Oprah, may urge you to do more yoga, as one reported benefit of the vegetable is increased joint flexibility. →→ *Preparation tip:* Robin's Fried Okra, courtesy of food writer Robin Carpenter: Rinse the okra and pat dry. Slice into ¼-inch rounds and dust in a mixture of cornmeal, corn flour, sea salt, and freshly ground black pepper. Heat 1 inch of either canola or corn oil in a frying pan until very hot. Drop the dusted okra into the oil and cook until browned, about 3 minutes. Remove and drain on paper towels. Serve immediately. (You can also take the same dusted okra and drop it into a lightly oiled, cast-iron skillet that is very hot and stir until the okra gets crunchy and slightly blackened.)

Olive Oil: This oil, carefully squeezed from the olive, makes tasty medicine. According to the Food and Drug Administration, 2 tablespoons of olive oil a day could help fight heart disease. Evidence suggests that olive oil's polyphenols promote heart health. Because polyphenols are easily destroyed, it is imperative to purchase the least-processed form of olive oil. The main fatty acid in olive oil, oleic acid, has been found to decrease the levels of cancer-causing genes associated with breast cancer. Oleic acid can also boost the effectiveness of cancer-fighting drugs. Packed with antioxidants, olive oil is believed to enhance absorption of vitamins D and E. Buyer beware: Olive oil that is labeled "100% pure" is often of the poorest quality—better-quality oils are labeled "Virgin." Avoid olive oil that is made with refined oils—this is a sure sign that the flavor and pH were chemically altered. You do want oils that say "Extra Virgin," "Cold Press," "Unfiltered," "Organic," and "Processed the same day as picked."

Food Sadhana

Make mealtime a sacred or honored event. Research indicates that you will maximize how you digest and assimilate food when you are relaxed. *Sadhana*, a Sanskrit word that means "practice," can describe a spiritual practice or an ordinary activity that is undertaken mindfully or with a focused purpose. That purpose can be to get more nourishment from food or to spend quality time with loved ones. When you practice eating and preparing food slowly, carefully, and with intention, you are practicing food sadhana. When you eat alone, avoid computer screens, televisions, and books. Focus on the moment and savoring the flavor and texture of your food. When eating with others, don't answer the phone or open a magazine. Perhaps spend the first five minutes with those at the table in silent appreciation of your meal. Slowing down and reducing stimulation from your environment during meals can help you digest more effectively and can contribute to a better spiritual and emotional connection with food.

Olives: Few people know that all olives are brined or pickled. Green olives are the same fruit as black olives, but less ripe. Olives are filled with monounsaturated fats, iron, vitamin E, and fiber. They are superb sources of oleic acid, an omega-9 monounsaturated fatty acid. Active compounds in olives have powerful anti-inflammatory properties that combat cancer and heart disease. Olives are flavorful antiaging pills filled with flavonoid polyphenols. For bonus health benefits, look for raw sun-dried olives or olives seasoned with sea salt and healing herbs.

Onion: Packed with the promise of good health, onions are members of the allium family. Pungent and full of sulfur-rich compounds that boost their disease-fighting arsenals, white, yellow, red, and sweet onions are used to add flavor to many dishes in cuisines around the world. Green onions and spring onions, or scallions, along with other varieties, are good sources of vitamin C, chromium, and fiber. The entire allium family, including garlic, leeks, and onions, is excellent for treating diseases prevalent in Western society, such as atherosclerosis, diabetes, and cancer. Onions are rich in one of the world's most powerful antioxidants, quercetin. Those suffering from arthritis and other degenerative diseases should eat raw or cooked onions to ward off inflammation. Onions contain the active inflammation-fighting compound called isothiocyanate, and this, plus vitamin C, quercetin, and flavonoids, makes onions worthy weapons against bacteria, especially during cold and flu season. And the list continues. Clinical research suggests that a sulfide in onions may be responsible for markedly lowering blood sugar after onion consumption. Chromium, a trace mineral that has been found to help cells respond to insulin, can be found in onions, making them a great food for diabetics. Onions have been flagged as an important food for heart health, significantly reducing the risk of heart disease in those who consume them regularly. Onions can lower unhealthy cholesterol and high blood pressure while also reducing the risk of heart attack. Adenosine found in onions inhibits blood clot formation. Onions have also been shown to have tumor-fighting capabilities. They also contain a newly discovered compound that inhibits the activity of osteoclasts and helps prevent bone loss, working similarly to the pharmaceutical drug Fosamax in helping to prevent the breakdown of bones. Ayurveda considers onions to be "tamasic," or slowing to the body and spirit. For similar reasons, onions are not eaten in certain temples in Japan, as they are thought to dull the mind. Because onions contain oxalate, those with kidney stones and gallbladder problems should avoid them.

Orange: Prepackaged in a protective rind, oranges are a bounty of flavonoids, vitamin C, and dietary fiber. Most people know that oranges contain large amounts of vitamin C, but few realize that vitamin C accounts for less than one-fifth of an orange's antioxidant power. Researchers have identified many lesser-known phytonutrients and flavonoids in oranges that account for the greater share of orange's free radical-fighting ability. Eating oranges can greatly reduce oxidative stress caused by free radicals, potentially slowing the process of aging and combating atherosclerosis and other degenerative diseases. Oranges are also a good source of potassium, folic acid, and B vitamins. Pectin, a fiber in oranges, can lower cholesterol levels. Don't forget the zest! The pith, or white part, of the orange is loaded with hesperidin, a key citrus flavonoid. In animal studies, hesperidin has been shown to lower cholesterol and blood pressure and to help fight inflammation. Eating oranges has been linked to reduced risk of cancer. Limonene, another citrus flavonoid, has been shown to be particularly effective in preventing and slowing the progression of lung cancer and breast cancer. Investigators found that limonene can cause cancerous cells to self-destruct.

Oregano: It's great on pasta, and it might help you beat a cold. Oregano's antibacterial compounds will battle an infection. It also eases muscle aches and pains and fights yeast inside and outside of the body. Many naturopaths recommended taking oregano internally as well as using oregano oil to fight athlete's foot.

Papaya: Sweet, tropical papayas contain an incredibly powerful enzyme, papain, that helps digest protein so effectively that, in some cases, it actually dissolves. Workers in papaya processing plants are required to wear protective gloves because lengthy exposure to papain will literally eat away at the flesh of their hands. Besides helping with indigestion, papaya may alleviate symptoms of diarrhea. In Chinese medicine, papaya will cool you off. A rich source of vitamin C, carotenes, flavonoids, and other antioxidants, papaya also contains potassium, folic acid, and vitamins A and E. Papaya's sunny color does more than brighten up your table—its carotenoids will save you from heart disease and cancer. ➤➤ *Preparation tip:* Eat fresh papaya with a traditional lime slice, or if the raw fruit is a little slimy for your taste, toss it in the blender with bananas, seasonal fruit, and water for a cleansing tonic. Or pick up papaya enzyme tablets at your local pharmacist.

Paprika: Paprika peppers have lycopene and vitamin C. They help stimulate circulation, regulate blood pressure, and fight bacterial infections. Sun-dried paprikas retain most of their healing phytochemicals, as opposed to paprika commercially processed at high temperatures. *See also* **Cayenne.**

Parsley: A superfood disguised as a mild-mannered green garnish, fresh parsley has a zesty flavor that even those who fear greens will enjoy. Ounce per ounce, parsley has more vitamin C than an orange, plenty of chlorophyll, folic acid, riboflavin, iron, and several minerals (magnesium, calcium, potassium, and zinc). Fiber, volatile oils, and flavonoids are all part of parsley. And what's in parsley is a lot of what's deficient in most standard American diets. Parsley is exceptionally high in many antioxidants, including vitamin C and carotenes that work as a team to lower the risk of cancer, heart disease, and stroke. Some of parsley's volatile oils and flavonoids have demonstrated unique cancer-fighting abilities. One particular volatile oil, myristicin, was shown to inhibit tumors in animal studies. Myristicin also works to activate an enzyme that cleans up oxidative stress. Garnish barbecue meats with fresh parsley, as it has been shown to neutralize benzopyrenes, the carcinogens formed in grilled or burnt meat and cigarette smoke.

Much of parsley's power can be found in the wisdom of ancient cultures. Chinese and German traditional medicine prescribed it to lower high blood pressure. Ancient Greeks and Romans used it as a digestive tonic and diuretic. It was used by members of the Cherokee tribe to strengthen the bladder. Juice enthusiasts believe that parsley will make you peppy and often include parsley in energy juices. Although many of parsley's cures are based in folklore, not hard science, there is no doubt that parsley supports the liver and kidneys and has a superb combination of antianemia nutrients. One ounce of parsley provides more iron than 8 ounces of pork. Folic acid in parsley helps build red blood cells, and its vitamin C improves iron absorption. As a powerful and palatable green that can be easily procured, supplement your life with a live food vitamin—parsley.

Parsnip: Cousin to the carrot, parsnips have a unique blend of potassium, phosphorus, sulfur, silicon, choline, and vitamin C, all good for the skin, hair, and nails. Parsnips were more popular than potatoes until the mid-nineteenth century. With a great deal more folate and dietary fiber than potatoes, there's good reason for parsnips to make a comeback. A diuretic, they detoxify the body and alleviate symptoms of arthritis. Parsnips and members of the carrot, or Umbelliferae, family contain phytonutrients that help combat cancer. Some of the most important of these compounds are phenolic acids that attach themselves to cancer-causing molecules and block them from being absorbed.

Passion Fruit: A tropical fruit mainly enjoyed for its juice, passion fruit has loads of vitamin C, phenolic acids, flavonoids, and carotenoids. Passion fruit is also a good source of vitamin A, potassium, and dietary fiber. Potassium in passion fruit supports healthy blood pressure levels, while phytochemicals in it support general cardiovascular health and cancer prevention. Studies at the University of Florida support passion fruit juice as a cancer-fighting substance.

Pawpaw; Papaw: Related to cherimoya (custard apple), pawpaw grows in the shade of the Mississippi Valley. Known as a true American native, pawpaw is one of the oldest indigenous fruits in the United States. Its popularity is building as organic growers realize how easy it is to cultivate this healthful fruit. Pawpaw grows without the need of pesticides; acetogenins contained in the tree's leaf, bark, and twig tissue are natural insecticides. In fact, these same acetogenins have demonstrated strong anticancer properties, preventing the spread of cancer cells in the body and controlling tumor growth. Nutrient-dense pawpaw contains plenty of vitamin C and minerals. It is high in protein and, compared to most fruits, also contains plenty of iron, copper, manganese, and adequate amounts of calcium, zinc, and niacin. ⇥ *Preparation tip:* Substitute pawpaw for any recipe calling for bananas.

Pea: Members of the pulse family, along with lentils and beans, peas have high levels of protein; are good sources of B vitamins, phosphorus, manganese, magnesium, potassium, and iron; and are an excellent source of the type of soluble dietary fiber that keeps blood sugar levels steady. For this reason, consuming peas can help keep mental concentration focused, lower blood cholesterol levels, and keep hunger at bay. Peas' fiber and ability to control blood sugar levels may help people to lose weight. Fresh peas are folate-rich, and some would say more appealing than other folate-rich veggies like watercress, spinach, or brussels sprouts. Fresh peas' vital nutrition is worth the effort of shucking them from their pods. ➤➤ *Preparation tip*: Add fresh raw or lightly steamed peas to salads or pasta dishes.

Peach: The heavenly sweet flavor of peaches and nectarines makes them a popular and coveted fruit. Fresh peaches are rich in potassium, carotenes, flavonoids, and natural sugars. Sink your teeth into the orange flesh and benefit from peaches' colorful phytochemicals. Lutein in nectarines and peaches protects against macular degeneration, heart disease, and cancer. ➤➤ *Preparation tip*: Slice up ripe peaches or nectarines and then sprinkle with raw cacao nibs. The crunch and bitter flavor blends well with the juicy sweetness of a peach, and your body will love you for eating this dessert.

Peanut: High in protein and monounsaturated fat (mainly oleic acid), peanuts are actually legumes. Antioxidants abound in peanuts, not to mention ample amounts of biotin, tocopherols, folic acid, magnesium, phosphorus, manganese, and vitamins B1, B3, and E. Although peanut allergies are common and can be severe, peanuts do have many health benefits, including cardio-protective features. One study showed that people who consumed a diet high in peanuts and peanut butter reduced their risk of heart disease by over 20 percent when compared to those who ate a standard American diet. Other studies showed that eating peanut products lowered cholesterol and triglyceride levels more than a low-fat diet. Peanuts also contain resveratrol, a phenolic antioxidant found in grapes and red wine. In clinical studies on animals, resveratrol has shown promise in cancer prevention and reversing cardiovascular disease. Many believe that consuming resveratrol in foods or in supplement form will help you live longer and healthier. Studies on living organisms including yeast, mice, and fish have demonstrated resveratrol's potential to extend life. Be aware that peanuts contain goitrogens that may become less active through cooking or roasting. Goitrogens should be avoided by those with pre-existing or untreated thyroid conditions. However, research remains unclear on the risk of peanut consumption on thyroid health. ⇥ *Preparation tip:* Not your usual circus treat, try some peanuts untouched by modern processing and growing methods. Delicious and unusual heirloom Amazonian Wild Jungle peanuts and Wild Jungle peanut butter are imported by raw food guru David Wolfe—see glossary for more information.

Pear: Sweet and juicy, pears are joyful fruits that provide vitamin C, potassium, and some folate. Their fiber stands out as their best feature—eat only one pear and you've eaten 25 percent of the suggested daily fiber intake. Soluble fiber in the form of pectin and lignin in pears helps absorb unhealthy cholesterol and clear it out of the digestive tract before it reaches the bloodstream. Pears come in many varieties, from Anjou to Red Bartlett, and their insoluble fiber helps things move smoothly through the intestines, thereby preventing constipation. Because high fiber intake is associated with reduced risk of colon cancer, those at risk for this degenerative disease would be wise to eat pears. ⇥ *Preparation tip:* For best results, eat pears with their skin on to get an optimum blast of fiber.

Persimmon: Greeks called persimmons fruit of the gods. An astringent fruit, persimmons are high in vitamin A, potassium, and fiber. They also contain several phytonutrients and the antitumor compounds betulinic acid and shibuol. The Fuyu variety has a firm consistency, like that of an apple. ➻ *Preparation tip*: If the common soft Hachiya variety of persimmons is too slimy or astringent for your taste, make a persimmon smoothie. Add one persimmon, an apple or a banana, and ½ to 1 cup water or ice or a combination. Blend until smooth and enjoy!

Pine Nut: Known for their starring role in pesto, these tiny flavorful nuts were once an important sustenance food for many Native American tribes, who enjoyed pine nuts' unusual texture, eating them whole or—to take advantage of their protein and fiber content—ground into wholesome soups, flours, and breads. We now know that pine nuts contain vitamin E; B vitamins 1, 2, and 3; as well as several minerals including iron, copper, magnesium, calcium, and manganese. In fact, as good sources of calcium and magnesium, pine nuts are calming to the mind and body. Pine nuts support a healthy heart and nervous system. ➻ *Preparation tip:* This is yet another healing food you can sprinkle on almost anything. Keep pine nuts on hand to add flavor to salads, pastas, soups, or even desserts.

Pineapple: Festive pineapple fills you up with plenty of vitamins C and B6, copper, and the magnificent micro-mineral manganese. A cofactor in critical enzymes that aid in the digestion and utilization of food, manganese also acts as a protective antioxidant. The remarkable phytonutrient bromelain, which is found in pineapple, stops inflammation and acts as a protein-digestive enzyme. In clinical trials, bromelain reduced swelling in acute sinusitis, sore throat, arthritis, and gout. Bromelain in pineapple seems to help dissolve uric acid. Pineapple's inflammation-fighting power may also help alleviate symptoms of carpal tunnel syndrome. Recommended for indigestion, pineapple helps reduce bloating in the last trimester of pregnancy, when digestion is most difficult. Slice up some fresh pineapple to decrease inflammation in your body or to help you digest a big meal. And don't forget, when you suffer from bronchitis or the flu, bromelain in pineapple can help break up mucous waste as you recover!

Pinto Bean: These beige beans with reddish-brown splashes of color have a similar nutritional profile to other common beans, such as black beans. Pinto beans support heart health by supplying almost three-quarters of the recommended daily amount of folate in one serving. Low in fat and high in protein, pinto beans are a good source of potassium and magnesium, both essential for healthy functioning of the cardiovascular system. The thiamine, or vitamin B1, contained in pinto beans supports energy and brain function. Pinto beans contain molybdenum, which fights the unhealthy effects of sulfites.

Plantain: *See* **Banana.**

Plum: Did you know there are over two thousand varieties of plums? Ranging in shade from purple to yellow, pink, green, and even orange, plums are packed with vitamin C and fiber. They have long been used as a cure for constipation. Dried plums are an even more effective laxative. Eat plums to prevent cancer and load up on antioxidants. They contain two related phenolic compounds—neochlorogenic and chlorogenic acid—that fight cancer and oxidative stress.

Pomegranate: Pumped full of disease-preventing antioxidants, pomegranates have been garnering a lot of attention for their healthy properties. Reports of pomegranate juice's protection against cardiovascular disease are making it a supermarket best seller. The fruit reduces oxidative stress that can lead to atherosclerosis. Research suggests that pomegranates and pomegranate juice can help alleviate symptoms of arthritis and fight many types of cancer. One study showed pomegranate joice may cut the harmful buildup of proteins linked to Alzheimer's disease. Antioxidants in pomegranate juice may also protect against the oxidative damage that leads to Alzheimer's. Traditionally used to alleviate diarrhea, too much pomegranate juice can make you constipated. ➤➤ *Preparation tip:* Susan Smith Jones writes this tip in her book, *The Healing Power of Nature Foods:* Fill a clean ice cube tray with pure pomegranate juice, freeze, and add to suitable beverages.

Pomelo: This fruit is similar to but less bitter than grapefruit. *See* **Grapefruit.**

Portobello Mushroom: Portobellos have all the health benefits of button mushrooms, but they taste meatier and have a higher protein content. Chunky and savory, portobellos are actually cremini mushrooms in size XXL. They make a good vegetarian entrée. *See also* **Mushroom.**

Potato: Unhealthy comfort food or healing food? Opinions are divided. In rushed and stressful times, perhaps we need potatoes' weightiness to slow us down. Undoubtedly, potatoes are heavy and difficult to digest, but they do have redeeming nutritional content, containing ample amounts of vitamins C, B6, niacin, and a healthy dose of fiber. Potatoes come in many sizes, shapes, and textures. A baked russet potato, eaten without the skin, has a higher glycemic index than baby potatoes eaten with the skin on.

In her book *The Jungle Effect*, Dr. Daphne Miller investigates traditional diets and their relationship to modern diseases. She examines the eating habits of Icelanders in regard to potatoes and finds that small, waxier potatoes are commonly consumed. As Miller discovered, these smaller, skin-rich potatoes have more nutrients and fiber than their larger counterparts, thereby preventing the usual spike in blood sugar that occurs with potato consumption. Small new potatoes encourage a healthier, more sustained release of energy. In Iceland many people boil enough potatoes for a week, which according to Miller also reduces the spuds' glycemic index as well. And what you put on the potato counts, too: Icelanders often enjoy potato salad with vinegar. As a condiment, vinegar can help moderate blood sugar levels and render foods like potatoes more easily digestible. Ayurveda recommends eating all potatoes with complementary, carminative spices like asafoedita, cumin, ginger, and black pepper. Hold the sour cream and enjoy the best that potatoes have to offer.

Propolis: Bees combine resin collected from leaves, buds, and bark of certain trees with enzymes and make it into propolis. Propolis contains vitamins, bioflavonoids, and amino acids, and has been found to build immunity especially in relation to fighting infection. Sold in Europe as a natural antibiotic, it can be used to fight common skin ailments and for dressing wounds and burns. Studies have shown it will kill or slow the growth of bacteria, viruses, and fungi.

Protein Powder: Protein powder may be made from whey, milk, egg, soy, peas, brown rice, or hemp. Because it is a processed food, ideally look for the least processed types. Use protein powders that haven't been heated, or at least not to very high temperatures. Don't use protein powders that have been chemically processed or produced. Stay as close to the original food as possible. Jennifer Cornbleet, author of *Raw Food Made Easy*, recommends Goatein Pure Goat's Milk Protein (Garden of Life) and Organic Hemp Protein Powder (Nutiva). *See also* **Whey Protein.**

Prune: Prunes have historically been used to alleviate constipation. While clinical studies of prunes' laxative abilities are lacking, many people have confirmed prunes' traditional reputation as an eliminator. Why not avoid over-the-counter chemical laxatives and give dried plums a try? Prunes contain phenolic compounds that have been shown to lower cholesterol. They also have plenty of antioxidants, vitamin A, potassium, and a significant ratio of fiber when compared to similar dried fruits like raisins. Some of the sweetness in plums comes from the unique natural sugar sorbitol. Prunes' glycemic index is rather moderate due to its sorbitol content. Two recent studies revealed that dried plums and dried plum bars elevated blood sugar slowly and provided sustained energy for athletes. In these studies, prunes compare favorably to Power Bars and other energy bars in providing steady fuel for athletic endeavors.

Psyllium Seed: Rich in dietary fiber, psyllium seeds have traditionally been used for their laxative powers. The key ingredient in Metamucil, psyllium seeds contain a gel-like fiber called mucilage, which can stop diarrhea, help lower cholesterol, and reduce the risk of heart disease and stroke.

Pumpkin: American colonists and Native Americans all ate pumpkins. Packed with carotenes and fiber, the pumpkin's rich orange color is the key to many of the healing plant compounds contained in this unique squash. Colorful carotenes in pumpkins help clean up damaging free radicals in the body. Lutein and zeaxanthin are carotenoids found in the lenses of the eyes that support vision health and prevent macular degeneration. Beta-carotene seems to offer protection from many types of cancer. Pumpkin's phenolic compounds seem to protect from potential cancers by binding carcinogens and blocking them from being absorbed by the body.

Pumpkin Seed; Pepita: Pumpkin seeds contain a great deal of zinc, magnesium, manganese, protein, and omega-3 oils. They also have plentiful supplies of iron, calcium, and phosphorus. Look to pumpkin seeds for vitamins E and B, especially niacin, monounsaturated fats, and phytosterols. One important phytosterol, beta-sitosterol, is known for being able to block conversion of testosterone into a substance that stimulates prostate enlargement. Several studies have shown evidence that ingesting pumpkin seed oil or beta-sitosterol improves symptoms of benign prostate enlargement. Zinc in pumpkin seeds seems to benefit prostate health as well. These findings back long-standing naturopathic recommendations for eating pumpkin seeds for prostate health. Phytosterols in pumpkin seeds have been shown to reduce overall unhealthy cholesterol levels, and you can pound down some pumpkin seeds for arthritis, too, as they have shown promise in some animal studies in reducing inflammation. Pumpkin seeds have also been a traditional remedy for intestinal parasites. ➼ *Preparation tip:* Save the seeds, whether you buy an organic pumpkin to carve or are cooking pumpkin meat. Rinse and remove the stringy insides of the pumpkin until all you have are seeds. You can eat these uncooked, dehydrated, or cooked at 225°F for 10 minutes.

Pumpkin Seed Oil: This oil adds flavor to salads or veggies and omega-3 fatty acids to your food—but do not heat it! Pumpkin seed oil omega-3 EFAs help to balance hormones, especially reproductive hormones.

Purslane: Rich in vitamins A, B, and C and stocked with iron, magnesium, and calcium, purslane has an illustrious history as a healing food. It was recommended for wound healing by Hippocrates, and Gandhi encouraged the people of India to grow purslane to foster self-sufficiency. Purslane, above all, is the best plant source of omega-3 essential fatty acids, holding close rank to flaxseeds and hemp seeds. Purslane can be found at Mexican produce stores and farmers markets or grown in colder climates. ↠ *Preparation tip:* Add a few handfuls of purslane to a soup or salad.

Quince: An astringent fruit with plenty of vitamin A, iron, and fiber, quince also contains many antioxidants and the mineral potassium. A bitter fruit that is related to apples and pears, quince is often served cooked or made into jellies or jams. Its potassium content keeps blood pressure levels steady. Quince contains tannins that boost the fruit's positive antioxidant profile and, like apples, contains quality fiber in the form of pectin. Eating quince fights free radicals, increases dietary fiber, and decreases your risk of cancer.

Quinoa (KEEN-wa): Closely related to amaranth, quinoa was called the mother grain by the ancient Incas. A staple in South America for thousands of years, it grows easily in the cold, high altitude of the Andes Mountains. With bragging rights as the grain with the most protein and more calcium than milk, quinoa's technically not a grain but the seed of a leafy plant. It flourishes in rough growing conditions, nourishing people whose environment can't sustain many other plant and animal foods. Quinoa's protein is good for vegetarians and vegans who need good plant-based sources of iron, calcium, and protein. More kudos for quinoa—its fiber and protein make it a low glycemic grain that keeps blood sugar levels steady. Quinoa also contains plenty of phosphorus, copper, magnesium, zinc, and vitamins B and E. Prepare it as a whole grain side dish, serve it as a salad, or buy it ground into flour for treats like gluten-free brownies. Traditional Chinese medicine recommends eating quinoa to strengthen the kidneys and revitalize the liver. Nutritionist Dr. Gillian McKeith recommends supercharging quinoa by sprouting the grain to unleash enzymes and activate phytonutrients.

Radicchio; Red Italian Chicory: Radicchio was cited in a famed Roman encyclopedia for its use as a blood purifier and tonic for insomniacs. Part of its bitter flavor is caused by intybin, a compound that acts as a sedative and blood purifier. Low in calories, chicory contains plenty of dietary fiber and vitamin C. One study in Italy identified radicchio as an underdog that came out on top in an antioxidant race, outscoring notoriously potent blueberries on the ORAC scale. Add radicchio to your longevity regime—it's a powerhouse of antiaging phytonutrients in the form of anthocynanins. *See also* **Chicory.**

Radish: A pungent root and member of the broccoli family, the radish has been used throughout history to treat liver ailments. Radishes' intense flavor is due to high levels of sulfur-based compounds, which help to increase the flow of bile, keeping the gallbladder and liver healthy and improving digestion. Radishes are an excellent source of vitamin C. Their greens contain even greater quantities of vitamin C, as well as calcium. Radishes are low in calories and high in fiber and water content. Daikon radishes are favored in Asian cuisines and contain additional copper and potassium. Macrobiotic dietary guidelines categorize daikons as yang in nature and helpful in purifying the blood. Red globes, common in North America, are high in the trace mineral molybdenum and are a good source of folic acid and potassium. Radishes help to dissolve mucus in the body and the digestive tract. They share the same cancer-stopping phytonutrients as their Brassica genus siblings, brussels sprouts, broccoli, and kale. ⤞ *Preparation tip:* Steam daikon radishes or add them sliced to soups.

Raisin: Considered a highly beneficial food in Ayurveda, raisins help raise your daily fiber intake and are a good source of plant-based iron. They also contain vitamins B1 and B6 and potassium. Many recommend raisins as a cure for constipation. One study showed that men and women who ate two or more servings of raisins a day had lower levels of bile acids and their food spent less transit time in the colon; both of these factors decrease the risk of colon cancer. Food science researchers have been investigating the use of raisins as a preserving agent in bacon, beef jerky, and lunch meats. These meat products are usually preserved with sodium nitrates, a compound that has been found to break down into cancer-causing chemicals in the human body. In a blind taste test, nitrate-free raisin jerky got the thumbs-up over chemically preserved jerky. ⇥ *Preparation tip:* Sprinkle sweet, sunshine-filled raisins on your cereal, yogurt, baked goods, or salads.

Rambutan: A close relation to the lychee, rambutan is a super supplier of flu-fighting vitamin C, as well as a sweet source of copper, manganese, and small amounts of important minerals like calcium and iron. Fresh rambutans look like a bright red sea urchins. Find them in Asian markets and specialty stores. Growing in popularity and more readily available are freeze-dried rambutans.

Raspberry: Related to roses and blackberries, these little pink jewels are low in calories and full of vitamin C and much more fiber than most fruits. They're not always pink—they come in yellow and other marvelous colors too. The insoluble fiber in raspberries makes them helpful for curing constipation, while their soluble fiber in the form of pectin helps lower unhealthy cholesterol levels. Raspberries contain the powerful cancer-busting phytonutrient ellagic acid. Replete with anthocyanins—the plant pigments that prevent cancer and heart disease—raspberries are a good weapon against many degenerative diseases. Delicate raspberries' hollow center makes them prone to spoil easily. Eat these berries fresh when in season or freeze for later use. ➤➤ *Preparation tip:* Add fresh raspberries to your salad.

Reishi Mushroom: A noted longevity food in Chinese medicine, reishi mushrooms are also used as a general tonic. Triterpenes in reishi mushrooms boost the immune system and have antiviral properties. Used to treat hepatitis B, reishi mushrooms are usually boiled in a broth or tea and then removed before consumption. *See also* **Mushroom.**

Homemade Rejuvelac

1. Soak 2 cups soft wheat berries in purified water 8 hours or overnight.
2. Drain, rinse, then allow to sprout for 2 days, without rinsing.
3. When white sprout tails begin to show, add 6 cups purified water, cover jar with cheesecloth, and put in a warm place where it can be exposed to at least 70°F temperatures for 2 days.
4. Pour off the water to drink, refrigerate, or use in a recipe. This is rejuvelac.
5. The leftover seeds can be used one more time, this time with 4 cups purified water, and the seeds will culture in 1 day. Then seeds can be composted or fed to the birds.

from Ann Wigmore Institute Kitchen,
Mary Forest Finnell, ND, MH, LMT

Rejuvelac: Created by health food pioneer Ann Wigmore, originator of the living food diet, rejuvelac is a fermented tonic rich in enzymes and believed to be cleansing for the intestines and colon. It provides good bacteria for the gut and intestinal system. Buy rejuvelac in health food stores or make your own.

Rhubarb: Rhubarb stalks contain a hefty percentage of insoluble fiber. Related to buckwheat, rhubarb's fiber is good for alleviating constipation. Bitter and acidic, it contains high levels of oxalates, which can cause stomach problems and kidney issues, so stay away from it if you have or have had kidney stones or gout. Look for fresh rhubarb with redder stalks if you prefer a slightly sweeter flavor. Rhubarb contains plenty of natural vitamin C, the antioxidant vitamin that naturally fights aging, heart disease, and macular degeneration. Rhubarb's insoluble fiber works similarly to oat and bran to clear the intestines of unhealthy cholesterol. Because of its bitter flavor, rhubarb is most often cooked and added to sweeter fruits like strawberries, but uncooked rhubarb can be an excellent choice. A German study tested raw vegetable juices for their cancer-preventative abilities, and rhubarb ranked close to number one in preventing cell mutations that often lead to cancer.

Royal Jelly: Bee pollen, honey, and enzymes are combined to make royal jelly—the thick liquid produced by worker bees to feed to developing bees, especially queen bees. A superfood for queen bees and for humans, royal jelly contains a plethora of vitamins, amino acids, and minerals. Recent medical research suggests that royal jelly has potential use as a cholesterol-lowering agent. It can also help prevent inflammation. As an adaptogen, it helps the body defend against chronic stress while building immunity and improving stamina.

Rutabaga: A cross between a turnip and kale. *See* **Turnip.**

Rye: A high fiber, gluten-free grain, rye has an intense flavor some people adore. A good source of phosphorus, magnesium, and vitamin B1, rye's fiber helps keep blood sugar levels steady. It has a combination of soluble and insoluble fiber that bulks up in the stomach and intestines when consumed, making one feel satiated. And as rye travels through the intestines, its fiber cleans out the digestive system. ↠ *Preparation tip:* Try baking with rye flour.

Sage: Antibacterial and anti-inflammatory properties in sage make it a good herb for many ailments. Often added for flavor, sage in sausage aids meat digestion. It has been cited for helping to improve mood and memory. Sage supports acetylcholine and keeps it from breaking down, thereby, many believe, helping prevent Alzheimer's disease.

Salt: Refined table salt is treated with chemicals and stripped of natural minerals. "Salt has the most grounding or descending activity of any substance used as food," explains Paul Pitchford, author of *Healing with Whole Foods.* In traditional Chinese medicine, natural sea or unrefined rock salt has a dual nature. Its yin side is calming, and its yang nature is believed to cause greed. Harvested from an ancient sea salt deposit, pink Himalayan sea salt is believed by some to be the purest salt on earth. Free from toxins, abundant in healing minerals, Himalayan pink salt has a delicious flavor and has been used therapeutically for thousands of years. Medical texts describe its use to heal wounds and to improve appetite. From an ancient seabed sealed with volcanic ash, Redmond's RealSalt is produced in the United States. Handselected and minimally processed, RealSalt comes from Redmond, Utah, and has a rich mineral content. People with high blood pressure swear RealSalt helps them keep their blood pressure in check. Unrefined sea salt contains the same blend of minerals found in the sea, including plenty of relaxing magnesium.

Used in traditional ceremonies, the sacred Hawaiian sea salt, Alaea is combined with mineral-rich Hawaiian clay to make a delicious and beneficial red salt. Evaporated by the sun and then combined with powdered lava and activated charcoal, Hiwa Kai is another traditional Hawaiian sea salt that can help the body safely release toxins. Its black color will add dramatic flair to your cooking. Truly unrefined salt is carefully harvested at low temperatures in locations like France, Hawaii, and Portugal. Most health food or gourmet shops carry a variety of sea salts from oceans and ancient seabeds around the world.

Seaweed: From the salty, mineral-rich waters of the sea comes a divine bounty. A true superfood, seaweed has the highest mineral content of any food substance on earth. Some varieties contain as much as ten times the amount of calcium as milk. All sea vegetables are rich in iodine, an essential mineral for the thyroid gland. Mineral ratios of the sea are nearly identical to the mineral profile of human blood, so sea vegetables contain this same mineral profile and are alkalizing to the blood. Eating seaweed arrests conditions of acidosis, or excess acid. Seaweed also contains cancer-protective lignans and algin, a colloidal carbohydrate, which reportedly attract various toxic metals and help the body safely pass them. Sea vegetables are not actually plants, but a form of marine algae that grows in the sunny parts of the ocean. Before being dried, most sea vegetables are 80 to 90 percent water. Once dried, seaweed is about 10 to 20 percent water. B vitamins and pantothenic acid in seaweed bust stress, while seaweed supports the cardiovascular system and beats inflammation. *See also* **Kelp**, **Kombu**, and **Dulse**.

Sesame Seed: Known in the Middle East as seeds of immortality, sesame seeds are rich in fat and more than 55 percent oil. Sesame seeds are about 20 percent protein and are high in minerals like zinc, copper, magnesium, phosphorus, and potassium as well as calcium. Sesame seeds contain vitamins A, E, and many B vitamins, as well as several phytonutrients. When added to grains and legumes, they offer amino acids, which make more complete proteins—especially helpful for vegetarians. Black sesame seeds are slightly higher in mineral content but have a more bitter flavor. Although sesame seeds are high in calcium, their high phosphorus content make them less than ideal for bone support because phosphorus must use calcium to be absorbed in the digestive tract. In Chinese medicine, sesame seeds fight deficiencies of the liver.

Unique lignans found in sesame seeds are sesamin and sesamolin. Both have demonstrated the ability to lower cholesterol and high blood pressure. In addition, sesamin has been shown to protect the liver from oxidative damage, backing sesame seeds' traditional use in Chinese medicine. Sesame seeds have as much iron as liver and also have two amino acids that are hard to come by in vegetable proteins—methionine and feel-good tryptophan. Unhulled sesame seeds contain far more calcium than hulled seeds, but the calcium in the hull comes in a form that is less absorbable for most people. Tahini is a creamy paste ground from hulled, raw, or roasted sesame seeds. Used to make hummus or baba ghanoush, tahini is also called sesame butter. Black sesame seed tahini is particularly nutritious. Remember that sesame hulls contain calcium oxalate and should be avoided by those suffering from gout or kidney issues.

Shallot: *See* **Onion.**

Shitake: Meaty, robust shitake mushrooms are symbolic of longevity in the East. Shitakes contain selenium, iron, protein, fiber, vitamin C, and other trace minerals. Lentinan in shitakes boosts immunity and fights infection, disease, and constitutional imbalances. Shitake mushrooms also contain eritadenine, a compound that can lower cholesterol levels. *See also* **Mushroom.**

Sorghum: The best grain you've never heard of, sorghum is widely consumed throughout Africa and Asia, where it has been cultivated as a staple grain for over four thousand years. Although relatively ignored in the West, sorghum is a gluten-free, antioxidant righ grain. Like corn, sorghum is a grass. It's an excellent supplier of dietary fiber, B vitamins (1, 2, and 3), iron, and potassium. What makes sorghum so special is that it's packed with healing phytonutrients like phenolic acids, flavonoids, and beta-glucans. Like colorful fruits and vegetables, darker sorghum varieties contain more antioxidants. Sorghum contains anthocyanins, also found in blueberries. Believe it or not, some varieties of sorghum contain more anthocyanins per gram than blueberries. Beta-glucans in sorghum are known for their role in immune system support and can have tumor-fighting properties. ⇥ *Preparation tip:* Similar to millet in texture, sorghum tastes better when toasted before cooking. It can be popped like popcorn, or make it into a soupy porridge. Cook with sorghum syrup, or use it to sweeten tea—it's like a healthier version of corn syrup.

Soy; Soybean: Cultivated in China for over thirteen thousand years, soybeans are one of the world's most widely eaten legumes. An excellent source of protein, they contain high levels of essential fatty acids, soy saponins, and isoflavones. Soybeans and traditional soy products have been an integral part of the diet in many Asian countries, especially Japan, China, and Korea, where soy products were traditionally processed and consumed. Today the United States is the largest grower and producer of soybeans and soy products. In 1999, the FDA approved labeling for soy products allowing manufacturers to declare soy beneficial for cardiovascular health. This led to soy's sudden surge in popularity and notoriety as a healthy food. However, most soy sold in the U.S. is very different from traditional soy foods. The careful processing and fermenting techniques of ancient times were cast aside for factory-produced tofurky, smart dogs, and soy bologna. A large percentage of U.S.-processed soy products use genetically modified soy beans. Decreasing consumption of animal proteins has many benefits including reduced risk of cardiovascular disease and many types of cancers. But when you reach for the fake bacon, make sure it's organic or at least labeled non GMO.

Soybeans have more phytic acid than any other bean. Phytic acid blocks the absorption of minerals, calcium, magnesium, iron, and zinc. Soybeans also inhibit the digestive enzyme trypsin, necessary for protein absorption. Fermented soybeans bypass trypsin inhibition and diminish the effects of phytic acid, another reason to try fermented soy foods such as tempeh, miso, and natto. Fermented soy products also support healthy intestinal flora and render soy easier to digest.

Isoflavones in soy are a class of phytoestrogens or plant compounds that mimic estrogenic activity in the body. How soy isoflavones imitate estrogen are dependent on many variables, including how the soy was processed. They may exert estrogenic and or anti-estrogenic effects in the human body. There are many conflicting opinions and studies on the positive and negative health effects of soy isoflavones and whether they are disruptive to the human endocrine system.

If you are concerned about the effects of soy protein, moderate consumption of soy would be most healthy, especially consuming only fermented or freshly prepared tofu and soy beans. Generally, avoid non-organic, commercially-produced soy products made with soy protein isolates, soy protein concentrates, hydrolyzed soy protein, and of course partially hydrogenated soy bean oil. *See also* **Edamame, Bean Curd, Miso,** and **Natto.**

Soup

A study at Pennsylvania State University found that soup helped slim dieters. Four hundred overweight men and women were put on calorie-controlled regimes and then divided into groups. The first group drank 10.5 ounces of soup as part of their daily diet. Group 2 sipped twice as much soup. Group 3 had no soup at all but consumed two dry processed snack foods. Group 4 was given no specific foods. A year later, those in group 2, who enjoyed two servings of soup a day, lost 50 percent more weight than all other groups.

Light and nourishing, soup is an important healing food in Ayurveda. It is often recommended for an easily digestible evening meal. In both traditional Chinese medicine and Ayurveda, it's important to adjust the diet to fit the seasons and even the time of day. Warm soup is very balancing during cold months and can be a great evening meal.

Both Ayurveda and traditional Chinese medicine recommend making soup fresh with high-quality produce, whole grains, soaked beans, and legumes.

Spelt: A much hardier grain than modern wheat, spelt has a sturdier hull that protects the grain from pollutants and pests. The hull is not removed until just before the grain is processed. Spelt doesn't have the same yield per acre as wheat, but those who choose spelt don't mind paying a little more for their health. It does have gluten, but it's much less allergenic than wheat, and it's more nutrient dense, with more protein, complex carbohydrates, and fiber. Spelt is also a good source of several B vitamins and minerals. Visionary and healer Hildegard of Bingen wrote about this hearty grain in the twelfth century: "The spelt is the best of grains. It is rich and nourishing and milder than other grain. It produces a strong body and healthy blood in those who eat it and it makes the spirit of man light and cheerful. If someone is ill boil some spelt, mix it with egg, and this will heal him like a fine ointment. Spelt grain makes body and blood healthy and the soul content."

Spinach: This nutrient-dense veggie has long had a reputation for increasing power and energy. Spinach has about twice as much iron as most other greens, not to mention vitamins C, E, and B, loads of folic acid, manganese, magnesium, calcium, and heaps of phytonutrients in your diet. Lutein in spinach is key in the prevention of macular degeneration. This green really shines in cancer prevention, as chlorophyll and carotene in spinach have been shown to keep cancer risk at bay. Researchers are so impressed by spinach's many cancer-preventing compounds, they went back to the lab. Further investigation indicated spinach extract slows stomach cancer and reduces skin cancer in mice. Spinach has also been related to a decrease in the incidence of breast cancer. Another notable nutrient in spinach is coenzyme Q10. An antioxidant that plays a critical role in energy production in every cell of the body, CoQ10 has been found to be beneficial in the treatment and prevention of many maladies, including allergies, Alzheimer's, and heart disease. CoQ10 has been flagged as an antiaging substance that aids circulation and revitalizes the immune system. And spinach could possibly cheer you up when you're down! Tyrosine, an amino acid in spinach, is needed for brain function and is directly involved in the production of vital neurotransmitters. A lack of tyrosine has been linked to mood disorders. But spinach contains purines and oxalates, so don't eat these greens if you suffer from gout or kidney stones.

Spirulina: *See* **Blue-Green Algae.**

Sprouted Wheat: Made from sprouted wheat berries that have been ground into flour, sprouted wheat bread has all the added benefits of being "sprouted." Activated enzymes in wheat sprouts make them a whole grain bread that's easier to digest. And protein, as well as added fiber, unlocked by the sprouting process gives sprouted wheat breads and baked goods a lower glycemic index than regular bread. Many people with wheat allergies or who have difficulty digesting wheat report no problem digesting sprouted wheat bread. More perishable than other baked goods, find sprouted wheat breads in the refrigerated section of your local health food store. *See also* **Sprouts.**

Sprouts: Sprouts are seeds, legumes, grains, or nuts that have been germinated into baby plants. They are made by soaking various seeds for three to five days until they have sprouted roots, tiny stems, or leaves. Because of their high concentration of vitamins, nutrients, enzymes, chlorophyll, protein, phytonutrients, and fiber, many categorize sprouts, especially certain ones, as superfoods. Sprouts are one of the most nutrient-dense and alkalizing foods. Dormant enzymes, proteins, nutrients, and phytochemicals are released when seeds sprout, and the human body seems to absorb vitamins from live sprouts much more readily. Protein in seeds, nuts, and grains increases by some 15 to 20 percent in sprout form. Sprouts help the body release accumulated acid waste and stimulate liver cleansing. Their activated enzymes boost digestion while their antioxidants fight stress. Sprouts have high concentrations of bioavailable B vitamins, adequate amounts of niacin, riboflavin, calcium phosphorus, iron, and vitamins C, E, and K.

In the study done at Johns Hopkins School of Medicine, broccoli sprouts were found to have thirty to fifty times the amount of anticancer compounds as the same amount of broccoli. Although not many studies have been done on sprouts, the broccoli sprout study and anecdotal reports about sprouts indicate they are a powerful medicine. Some of the most common sprouts are alfalfa, sunflower, and mung. Other sprouts include pumpkin, sunflower, sesame, mustard, fenugreek, radish, buckwheat, clover, quinoa, millet, rye, corn, rice, oats, barley, spelt, amaranth, Kamut, almond, cashew, hazelnut, Brazil nut, pine nut, pecan, pistachio, walnut, lentil, adzuki bean, kidney bean, navy bean, or green peas. Microgreens are sprouts too! Grown upright, these sprouts are cultivated in light as opposed to other sprouts that lie in dark moisture to germinate. As a result, microgreens look more like mini plants, but there is nothing small about their nutritional content. Argula microgreens have the same nutritional benefits as argula—concentrated. ⇥ *Preparation tip:* Purchase sprouting equipment at your local health food store or online. *See also* **Alfalfa Sprouts.**

Star Fruit: Rich in antioxidants and vitamin C, yet low in sugar, star fruit has a pleasantly sweet flavor. A good source of vitamin A, fiber, and potassium, its unusual shape when cut crosswise makes a beautiful presentation on a plate. Grown in Florida and Hawaii, this tropical fruit is traditionally used as a diuretic. In China, star fruit juice is used to clean temples. One of the few fruits that contain calcium, star fruit also contains amino acids, phosphorus, riboflavin, and antioxidants. Do not eat star fruit or star fruit products if you suffer from kidney stones or gout, as they contain oxalic acid. And check with your doctor if you are on certain prescription medications, such as statins or benzodiazepines, as star fruit contains powerful enzyme inhibitors that diminish the effectiveness of these drugs.

Stevia: A sweet leaf that belongs to the chrysanthemum family and originated in Paraguay, stevia was used by the Guarani Indians to sweeten tea, aid digestion, and dress wounds. Sweet stevia contains compounds called glycosides that are sweet but can't be absorbed by the body. Stevia also contains protein, minerals, vitamins A and C, and provides a sweet flavor to foods without elevating blood sugar. Studies suggest it actually keeps blood sugar levels steady in diabetics and pre-diabetics. Stevia does not encourage yeast and bacterial growth like conventional sugar; it has been shown to inhibit the growth of *Streptococcus mutans*. Preliminary studies have indicated that stevia may be of help for people who suffer from high blood pressure. Stevia has zero calories and a zero glycemic index.

Strawberry: High in vitamins C and K, manganese, fiber, and flavonoids, strawberries are filled with a powerful phytonutrient that gives them their bright red color: anthocyanidin. Scientific studies reveal the anthocynadins in strawberries seem to block an enzyme called cyclooxygenase (COX) that causes inflammation. Blocking cyclooxygenase enzymes sounds complicated, but it's the same thing you block when you take an aspirin or ibuprofen to stop inflammation. Not many people are aware of the potential of strawberries as COX inhibitors. Studies also link a diet that contains strawberries to lower death rates from cancer. There is no direct scientific evidence, but the fact that strawberries contain the cancer-attacking phytonutrient ellagic acid seems to be the reason. ⇥ *Preparation tip:* Most of us know what to do with fresh strawberries but not the best way to store them. When you bring them home from the grocery store or farmers market, immediately place them in an airtight container layered with paper towels. Put the container in the fridge for up to a week. Wait to wash the berries until immediately before you eat them. Freezing berries doesn't destroy their phytonutrient content.

Sucanat: A brand of unrefined whole cane sugar, Sucanat retains the mineral salts, trace elements, and part of the vitamins and vegetable fibers found in the sugarcane plant.

Summer Squash: Related to melons, summer squash retains more water than other squash, therefore making it more hydrating and balancing in summer months. In laboratory investigations focused specifically on summer squash juices, the liquid was shown to prevent cell mutations. *See also* **Zucchini.**

Sunchoke: *See* **Jerusalem Artichoke.**

Sunflower Seed: Sunflower seeds contain many nutrients that are typically lacking in a Western diet. For this reason many naturopathic doctors recommend snacking on these satisfying seeds. High in vitamin E, magnesium, selenium, phosphorus, copper, iron, folic acid, and vitamins B1, B5, and B6, they were cultivated and enjoyed for over five thousand years by indigenous people of North and South America. Sunflower seeds have the same beneficial properties as most nuts and seeds. They are particularly unique in their high content of the mineral selenium, which has demonstrated clear anticancer, anti-inflammatory, and anti-allergenic properties. Sunflower seeds provide a whopping 75 percent of the USRDA of vitamin E, a powerful antioxidant vitamin and anticancer agent in its own right. Delicious on salads and sandwiches, sprouted sunflower seeds offer the same benefits turbocharged. ↠ *Preparation tip:* Grab portable sunflower seeds and eat a handful for a quick snack on the go. British nutritionist Dr. Gillian McKeith advises sunflower seeds "are far better for you than a cup of coffee or some snack foods that simply give you a zap of sugar, and excess calories." *See also* **Sprouts.**

Sweet Potato: According to the ancient healing tradition of Ayurveda, sweet potatoes have the powerful ability to literally root us back to who we are when we are confused, tired, scattered, or out of balance. Scientifically, sweet potatoes are tubers that are an excellent source of carotenes and vitamins C and B6. With far more nutrients than the more popular white potato, sweet potatoes are a good source of vitamin E and minerals manganese, copper, and biotin. Sweet potatoes also have a lower glycemic index than white potatoes and actually help stabilize blood sugar, making them a healthy food for diabetics. ⇥ *Preparation tip:* Make sweet potato fries. Slice ½- to 1-inch strips of sweet potatoes and then spray or coat lightly with cooking oil. Bake in the oven at 425°F for 12–14 minutes.

Swiss Chard: Instead of nasal spray, ancient Greeks and Romans used Swiss chard as a decongestant. Heavily stocked with vitamins, it is an excellent source of vitamins C, E, and K, as well as fiber and chlorophyll. Chard also contains minerals, magnesium, potassium, iron, manganese, and calcium. Swiss chard has been found to be a good weapon against many types of cancers, especially colon cancer. It has almost 400 percent of the USRDA of vitamin K, which activates osteocalcin, a protein that works like glue to stick new calcium molecules to the bone—making Swiss chard an excellent food for bone health.

Tahini: *See* **Sesame Seed.**

Tamarind: The fruit of the tamarind has a brown pod. Inside are hard seeds and a pulp used in traditional cooking around the world. In the West, a popular dish that features the unique sour, acidic flavor of tamarind is the Thai noodle dish pad thai. A source of vitamin C, fiber, potassium, and magnesium as well as smaller quantities of several other nutrients, tamarind has numerous reported medicinal properties in the countries where its use is prevalent. It is often utilized to reduce fever, and its vitamin C content may protect against colds. Also known to help with digestion with mild laxative effects, tamarind has a multitude of antioxidants that may be protective against cancer. ⇥ *Preparation tip:* Look for tamarind paste or fresh pods through gourmet or ethnic grocers. Many grocers like Trader Joe's sell easy-to-prepare box mixes of pad thai—add fresh ingredients like cilantro, mung bean sprouts, and a little fresh tamarind or tamarind paste, along with other ingredients to make a quick and easy antioxidant-rich dish.

Tangerine; Tangelo; Tangor: *See* **Orange.**

Tapioca Flour: *See* **Yucca.**

Taro: Toxic in its raw form due to high levels of oxalates, taro must be soaked overnight to eliminate oxalic acids. Though grown around the world, fresh taro is hard to find in the United States, unless of course you're in Hawaii. The Hawaiian Islanders believed taro had divine powers. Often made into a thick, slightly fermented paste called poi, taro is most often sold in chip form on the mainland. As a healthier kind of potato chip, taro chips can slightly boost your daily calcium, vitamin C, and iron content.

Tea: *Camellia sinensis* can be surprisingly delicious to eat. A Burmese restaurant in San Francisco makes a delicious tea salad that features a few teaspoons of steeped green tea. And tea contains L-theanine, a stress-busting amino acid that seems to counter the effects of caffeine and in turn may decrease appetite. You also catch something called a catechin when you eat tea with your food. A polyphenol, catechin is part of a powerful group of antioxidants. Scientists studying the polyphenols found in tea discovered that they seem to work in unison with caffeine to stimulate thermogenesis, or the process by which the body burns fat to produce energy. Catechins also appear to houseclean the blood of triglycerides, which play a part in elevating cholesterol. All caffeinated tea comes from the plant *Camellia sinensis*—the difference in teas is all in the processing. Look below for more info on your favorite tea.

White Tea: The tea of royalty—sweet and sublime—white tea is the least processed and is packed with flavonoids that rescue us from the ravages of free radical damage.

Green Tea: This highly publicized healthy tea undergoes minimal oxidation and has less caffeine than black tea. Green tea heals through antioxidant power.

Oolong Tea: The leaves of oolong tea are mildly fermented to give them a smoky flavor that lends well to cooked dishes.

Black Tea: Black tea leaves are oxidized the longest and have the most caffeine, but they still contain plenty of polyphenols.

Brew up a cup, save the leaves, and add them to your soup, salad, or stir-fry. For further recipes and information, read *Cooking with Tea* by Robert Wemischner and Diana Rosen.

Teff: From Ethiopia comes this ancient grain so small its name means "lost." Used to make a sour, spongy bread called inerja, teff is loaded with calcium, iron, protein, and magnesium. It is also an excellent source of amino acids. It's very high in fiber for a grain—it's too small to shed its endosperm—so it's always a "whole grain." Look for gluten-free teff or teff flour in health food stores.

Tempeh: A staple food in Indonesia for over 2000 years, tempeh is a traditionally-processed soy food. Hearty in flavor and high in protein, it makes a delicious vegan meat substitute. Because tempeh is made by fermenting soy beans, it contains antibiotic agents and enzymes that make soy easier to digest. Many consider tempeh and other fermented soy foods superior for these reasons. It has isoflavones and soy saponins that bestow healing benefits like decreased risk of heart disease and protection against some cancers. And because tempeh is rich in dietary fiber, it's a great protein for diabetics for whom animal proteins are problematic. It's rich in manganese, riboflavin, and magnesium.

Tofu: *See* **Bean Curd.**

Tomato; Tomatillo; Cherry Tomato: The popular tomato is almost 90 percent water. Tomatoes come in many varieties and have been called a superfood, mostly because of their high lycopene content. This unique phytonutrient has many known curative effects that have been extensively documented in various scientific studies. Tomatoes also contain ample amounts of vitamins C, B6, niacin, folate, thiamine, and pantothenic acid, and minerals potassium, chromium, biotin, lutein, zeaxanthin, and alpha and beta-carotene. The aforementioned lycopene is not only a key healing ingredient but also the carotenoid responsible for tomato's red color. Tomato's total package of nutrients and antioxidants can help raise the body's natural sun protection factor. Lycopene-laden tomatoes have also been cited in many studies that demonstrate eating lots of tomatoes decreases the risk of many forms of cancer, especially prostate cancer. Tomato's lycopene content may also benefit the heart, helping prevent heart disease. ⤏ *Preparation tip:* Lycopene in cooked tomatoes is slightly more absorbable than in raw tomatoes. The skin of tomatoes is the most nutrient-dense part, so don't peel it. Better yet eat cherry tomatoes when in season, as these tiny tomatoes have the most skin, healing antioxidants, and nutrients.

Healthy Fats Could Promote Weight Loss

Dr. Gillian McKeith tells her clients to call essential fatty acids "essential skinny acids." She wants to remind those in her care that EFAs have been shown to help you lose, rather than gain, weight. It may be because they are used in every cell of your body. If you are low on EFAs, your body will use whatever fat is available and keep sending the brain signals to eat more fat. Cell membranes are comprised of EFAs. Western diets have an abundance of some omega-6 fatty acids, yet we need a balance of omega-3s and omega-6s. Omega-3 oils are the most volatile oils, and they add fluidity to the cell membrane. If the body lacks adequate amounts of omega-3 oils, the cells will use any other fats available to maintain the integrity of the cell walls. But cell membranes made from incorrect fats may be rigid or leaky. Many health care providers recommend consuming more foods rich in omega-3 oils. When buying fresh oils rich in omega-3s, such as walnut oil, flax oil, pumpkin seed oil, fish oil, cod liver oil, and hemp seed oil, be sure to purchase them cold pressed and check the expiration date. One of the reasons omega-3s were replaced by other oils in processed foods is that they deteriorate quickly, especially in warm weather. A shorter shelf life means less profitability for large manufacturers.

Tulsi: Indian basil, tulsi, comes in three varieties: Krishna, Rama, and Vana. A sacred herb that Ganesh wears as a garland around his neck, tulsi is revered in Indian medicine.

Tulsi has been studied scientifically and experientially for thousands of years. Indian people keep holy basil plants in their homes for good luck and to purify the air. Classified as an adaptogen, tulsi helps the body deal with the adverse effects of stress and builds immunity without any side effects. Tulsi has an abundance of antioxidants and may help regulate blood sugar. Tulsi will help ward off colds and may be more effective than a flu shot. Most often prepared as a tea, it can also be taken in a pill form or grown in warm climates and used to flavor foods. Use fresh tulsi like Italian basil.

Turmeric: A root, or rhizome, related to ginger, turmeric is most often dried and used as a spice. Turmeric's main active agent, curcumin, reduces the chance of stroke and is a natural inhibitor of enzymes that cause inflammation. In fact, so incredible is turmeric as a plant-based anti-inflammatory agent, it rivals many prescription anti-inflammatory drugs. Curcumin gives turmeric its brilliant yellow color—so powerful, it's used to dye clothing in Asia. Turmeric's bitter flavor blends well in curries, and its list of healing properties seems endless. Studies confirm its remarkable anticarcinogenic abilities. One found that a combination of cruciferous vegetables and turmeric were more powerful at fighting prostate cancer when combined than when taken separately. The growing number of people suffering from inflammatory bowel diseases can turn to seasoning foods with turmeric—studies on animals show that when consumed, tumeric improved intestinal cell function and reduced inflammation associated with digestive disorders. Turmeric guards against Alzheimer's by triggering a protective system that is believed to stop the oxidation responsible for dementia. Research suggests that turmeric can help the liver detoxify from carcinogenic chemicals and improves overall liver function. Turmeric is a powerful ally in the battle against heart disease. It helps prevent the oxidation of cholesterol in the body that leads to atherosclerosis. India, a country that consumes copious amounts of turmeric, has the lowest rates of breast and prostate cancer, Alzheimer's, and other age-related, degenerative diseases, in the world. Sometimes the root can be found fresh and can be used like ginger, sliced and sautéed in curries and stir-fries.

Turnip: Another cruciferous vegetable, sometimes considered a starch, turnip roots have only one-third the calories of a baked potato and far more fiber. Benefits of eating turnip roots include getting plenty of vitamin C, folic acid, pantothenic acid, and manganese. Turnip greens, like most greens, are extremely nutrient dense and high in vitamins C, B6, E, and folic acid. Greens from turnips are rich suppliers of minerals including calcium, copper, and manganese. ⇸ *Preparation tip:* Serve mashed turnip root for a fiber-rich, low-calorie potato substitute. Make it just like potatoes. Peel, boil, or steam, and then mash. *See also* **Broccoli**, **Cabbage**.

Vanilla: Vanilla is the edible fruit of a tropical orchid. Mexican royalty used vanilla as an aphrodisiac, and one study showed that men responded to the aroma of vanilla. Vanilla was used by indigenous people to calm an upset stomach. The less processed the vanilla, the better, so purchase whole pods or pure vanilla in the form of raw powder or extract for your recipes.

Vinegar: Made with a two-step fermentation process, there are a multitude of vinegars available, from the artisanal to the ordinary. In the first step of vinegar production, sugar, fruit juice, honey, and molasses are fermented into alcohol. In the second stage, naturally occurring bacteria known as acetobaters are combined with the alcohol to form acetic acid, the substance that gives vinegar its sour flavor. Not much formal research has been done on vinegar, but it has been used as a folk remedy for many ailments. Experts do agree that acetic acid helps the body absorb minerals, making vinegar an important seasoning for women who have difficulty assimilating calcium. It also controls blood sugar. Investigators believe that it may inactivate some of the digestive enzymes that break down carbohydrates into sugars, slowing down sudden spikes in blood sugar. ⇥ *Preparation tip:* Explore the gastronomic delights of exotic vinegars! Try dressing your next salad with a little olive oil and aged balsamic or champagne vinegar . *See also* **Apple Cider Vinegar.**

Wakame: A brown sea vegetable, wakame contains fucoxanthin, calcium, iron, natural sodium, and a bit of vitamin C. Fucoxanthin, an edible carotenoid in brown seaweed, has many potential benefits that are currently under investigation. Japanese researchers found fucoxanthin helped animals lose 10 percent of their body weight. And even more significant is the role fucoxanthin is believed to play in increasing the rate at which abdominal fat is burned, something many people would love some assistance with. *See also* **Seaweed, Kombu.**

Walnut: Nutrient-rich walnuts are an excellent vegetarian source of omega-3 oils. As one of the only nuts that contain omega-3s, walnuts are also the main non-fish source of alpha-linolenic acid. Studies have specifically pointed out walnuts for their role in reducing unhealthy cholesterol. Arginine, an amino acid in many nuts, supports healthy and flexible veins. Ellagic acid, an antioxidant present in walnuts, acts as a defender against cancer and heart disease by blocking metabolic pathways that contribute to the development of these devastating diseases. ⇥ *Preparation tip:* Because walnuts are high in volatile fatty acids, make sure you buy raw walnuts for their omega-3 oils. Keep fresh walnuts in the freezer or fridge to prevent oils from going rancid.

Water Chestnut: Not nuts but roots that grow from an aquatic rush grass, water chestnuts are high in potassium and fiber. Traditionally, water chestnuts have been used to cure indigestion and nausea. Look for fresh water chestnuts in Asian specialty stores, or purchase more widely available canned water chestnuts.

Watercress: Low in calories, watercress is a good source of iron, calcium, phosphorus, potassium, and vitamins A, K, and C. Watercress also contains lutein and beta-carotene. It seems to protect smokers from lung cancer by inhibiting a potent carcinogenic in tobacco. Reportedly, watercress aids digestion and acts as a diuretic. ➻ *Preparation tip:* Purchase a bundle of watercress. Wash and remove the usually soil-laden roots. Keep in a bag with a paper or cloth napkin to soak up excess moisture. During the week, add watercress to salads, sandwiches, soups, and other cooked foods to increase your intake of raw greens!

Watermelon: Watermelon is 90 percent water, making it a juicy fruit and a natural diuretic, perfect food for a hot summer's day. In fact, watermelon seems made by Mother Nature to cool heat-related illnesses. It contains vitamins C and A as well as potassium and many powerful antioxidants. Watermelon is good for edema and lowering blood pressure naturally. ➻ *Preparation tip:* Fresh juiced watermelon is a tremendously alkalizing and healing drink. Juice expert Steve Meyerowitz advocates juicing not only the watermelon meat, but also the rind and even the seeds, thereby releasing an array of therapeutic plant compounds that reoxygenate the cells and scavenge for free radicals.

Wheat Germ Oil: One of the richest food sources of vitamin E, wheat germ oil in the diet provides this important antioxidant vitamin.

Wheatgrass: Very high in chlorophyll, wheatgrass can be juiced fresh or taken as a dried powder. Rich in many vitamins and minerals, wheatgrass has as much calcium per ounce as milk and plenty of iron, vitamin C, sodium, potassium, and magnesium. Wheatgrass has a high protein content and hundreds of unique digestive enzymes, including the powerful antioxidant superoxide dismutase, or SOD. Wheatgrass has been reported to help keep eczema at bay, prevent tooth decay, build blood, cleanse the liver, slow down aging, and help maintain steady blood sugar levels. Those allergic to wheat are rarely allergic to its grass stage. Fresh wheatgrass is most effective because it contains live enzymes that are not present in dried or powdered form. Minimally processed, organic, low-temperature dried wheatgrass juice makes a great runner up.

Whey Protein: For those looking for more protein in their diet, whey protein is a form that's easy to absorb. There are many whey protein powders on the market, so don't fire up your blender until you know the facts. Whey is formed from the liquids that separate from the curd in the cheese-making process. Raw whey is rich in varied protein compounds known as microfractions. Many of these protein fractions have great health benefits; unfortunately, many are diminished, destroyed, or damaged in processing. Exposure to heat also affects the protein fractions in whey. Many of the different protein fractions found in whey can be easily absorbed. Others support immunity and have antioxidant, cell protective, antibacterial, and antimicrobial properties. For these reasons, whey protein is often heralded as a health-boosting food. However, the world of whey protein can get complicated. Whey protein usually comes in three different types: Concentrate, Hydrosolate, and Isolate. Isolate whey protein is the best and most expensive whey protein because it is most like the whole food. It will ideally have the word *undenatured,* meaning the healing protein fractions have not been denatured or altered in processing. Whey protein concentrate is the most highly processed, so it costs less than other forms. Try to avoid it. Hydrolyzed whey protein is pre-digested or treated with enzymes to break down the amino acid chains. Because some people are allergic to protein fractions, this form of whey is hypoallergenic. However, in breaking down protein fractions, proteins are changed from their natural, whole food form. Ion-exchanged protein is separated through electrical charge, causing dramatic changes in pH that destroy several whey protein fractions. Some fractions survive. ➺ *Preparation tip:* Whey is a dairy product, so those allergic to dairy should steer clear of undenatured whey protein. And whey should be made from the milk of cows not treated with rbGH.

Wild Rice: Native to the Great Lakes region of North America, wild rice was a staple food for many Native Americans. Members of the Menominee tribe called it "the precious grain sent by The Great Spirit to serve as food." Although it looks like rice, it's actually a marsh grass seed. Wild rice is low in fat and sodium and high in protein, fiber, B vitamins, phosphorus, and potassium. There are many varieties of wild rice, including hybrids cultivated in California, Idaho, and Canada. ⇥ *Preparation tip:* Add wild rice to soups or stews or blend it with other rice dishes.

Winter Squash: This category encompasses several varieties of squash loaded with vitamin A, including acorn, buttercup, butternut, calabaza, hubbard, pumpkin, and spaghetti squashes. *See also* **Pumpkin.**

Xylitol (ZIGH-le-tol) : A naturally occurring sugar alcohol, xylitol can be extracted from the plant fiber of birch trees, raspberries, plums, corn, and various other fruits and vegetables. Xylitol was popularized by Finnish producers in the 1960s who extracted xylitol from birch trees and advertised it as a sweetener that was safe for diabetics. Low in calories compared to white sugar, xylitol also has a substantially lower glycemic index than sugar, making it a good choice for diabetics and others with blood sugar issues. A tooth-friendly sugar, xylitol also has plaque-reducing effects, as confirmed by research. It seems to attract and then starve microorganisms like yeast and bacteria, and it also prevents bacteria from adhering to the walls of the sinuses and upper respiratory tract. Finnish research suggests that xylitol may have potential for treating osteoporosis, as some studies have demonstrated that bone density in rats increased when they consumed xylitol. Don't bake yeast bread with xylitol or its yeast-killing ability will keep the bread from rising. And beware of leaving xylitol out around your pet pooch—it is harmless for humans but can be fatal for dogs. Look for xylitol in the supplement section of your health food store—the USDA has classified it as a food additive even though you can use it just like sugar.

Yacon Syrup: A low-glycemic sweetener, yacon syrup is derived from the yacon plant, indigenous to South America. Yacon syrup contains the world's richest source of fructooligosaccharides, or FOS, long-chain sugars that encourage the growth of healthy bacteria in the gut. Use yacon syrup as a healthy, low-glycemic sweetener.

Yam: A great food for the ladies, yams are high in vitamin B6, which assists the liver in detoxifying excess estrogen. Yams are also a good source of dietary fiber and potassium. A unique phytoestrogen in yams, diosgenin, is a phytochemical used in the synthesis of pharmaceutical progesterone. One double-blind study concluded that women suffering from PMS and fibrocystic breasts had relief from symptoms when vitamin B6 was taken.

Yogurt: Because it's fermented, yogurt is easier on the digestive system than most other dairy foods. Filled with probiotics, or healthy bacteria, yogurt helps to prevent yeast infections. It's a good idea to eat yogurt after you've had a dose of antibiotics because all bacteria, including beneficial bacteria get destroyed by prescription antibiotics. Yogurt made from goat, cow, or sheep milk helps build friendly flora in the intestinal tract. A study done at University of California, Davis, supports the theory that yogurt boosts immunity. People who ate two cups of yogurt a day for four months tested higher in gamma interferon—a protein that supports the work of white blood cells—than those who had no yogurt. A great source of calcium, whole milk yogurt is less processed than the often recommended non- or low-fat yogurt.

Today, many premium and artisanal yogurts are made from the milk of grass-fed cows. Although this yogurt comes with a higher price tag, it invariably provides more healthy omega-3 fatty acids.

Yucca; Cassava; Manio: A starchy, tuberous root, yucca is the world's number-two vegetable crop, just behind potatoes. Most well-known in the West for its role as the main ingredient in tapioca, this tropical root is used to make an incredibly diverse variety of regional dishes, from fermented soup to empanadas. Yucca is a dietary staple in Africa, Asia, South America, and the Caribbean, but the United States seems to be the last to know about the healing potential of one of the world's most famous foods. Yucca has plenty of iron, vitamin C, and magnesium, making it great for women of childbearing age and growing children. Imagine telling the kids, "We'll be having mashed yucca tonight!" But you'll be setting them on an early start to a healthy life. Yucca's high vitamin C content is good for all ages and is especially protective against cancer, heart disease, and cataracts. One study in the Philippines examined an array of fiber-rich roots and legumes. Of the twelve roots and beans, which included sweet potatoes, peanuts, and kidney beans, yucca came up number one for reducing unhealthy LDL cholesterol. For those with wheat allergies, cassava flour, or tapioca flour, is a gluten-free alternative to wheat flour. Find tapioca flour at most health food stores or gourmet grocers. Acquiring a fresh manioc tuber may require more work. Search for yucca (you may have to ask for manioc or cassava) at ethnic or gourmet grocers. ⇥ *Preparation tip:* For whole yucca, think like you're cooking a potato. First, peel the yucca, and then cut it into 2- or 3-inch pieces. Slice each piece lengthwise and remove the tough inner fiber that runs down the middle. Boil or steam, mash, garnish, and serve like you would a potato.

Zucchini; Summer Squash; Squash Blossoms: Eat your zukes! Zucchini, especially raw, has a mildly diuretic effect. It will fill you up without a lot of calories. Over 75 percent water, delicious, fiber-rich zucchinis provide plenty of vitamins A and C, potassium, and iron. Naturally low fat, one serving is only 25 calories. Add zucchini to your diet for phytonutrient power and to help you build up defenses against degenerative diseases, especially cancer. Zucchini is a summer squash that helps the body deal with heat by hydrating it. Carotenes in summer squash help to protect skin from sun damage.

What to Eat: Ailment Treatment and Health Maintenance

Diet, exercise, and lifestyle are recognized as key components to overall health and well-being. Most ancient societies recognized the importance of eating and utilizing the medicinal foods available to them. Recovery, prevention, and alleviation of symptoms of degenerative diseases can be augmented with a healing foods diet. The importance of working with an expert to select optimum foods should not be underestimated. Use the guide below to help make healthy choices for you and your family. In the case of diagnosed conditions or diseases, always check with your doctor when using foods or diet as a part of your overall treatment program.

ADD; Attention Deficit Disorder: Avoid processed foods, sweets, and sodas. *See also* **Brain Function and Memory** and **Calming Foods**.

Acid/Alkaline Foods: To maintain a healthy pH, in general, consume 80 percent alkaline-forming foods and 20 percent acid-forming foods. The term *pH* means "potential of hydrogen" and measures acidity through hydrogen activity in water—which is made up of two hydrogen atoms and a larger oxygen atom. Normal pH should be slightly alkaline at 7.25.

In general, acid-forming foods are flesh proteins, dairy, tea, wine, coffee, and soft drinks. A partial list of acid-forming foods includes: beer, buckwheat, butter, catsup, cranberries, eggs, fish, legumes, meat, milk, olives, pasta, prescription medications, processed foods, poultry, shellfish, sugar, soft drinks, tea, vinegar, wine.

The most alkaline-forming foods are fresh raw fruits and veggies. A partial list of alkaline-forming foods includes: avocados, broccoli, corn, coconut, dates, fresh fruits and veggies, honey, horseradish, maple syrup, mushrooms, onions, sea vegetables, spinach, sprouts, and watercress.

Acid Reflux: cranberries, cranberry juice, okra, meals eaten slowly, foods high in dietary fiber. Make an apple cider vinegar drink of 8 ounces water mixed with 1 tablespoon raw, unfiltered apple cider vinegar, and add honey or sweeten to taste. Avoid processed foods, excess animal products, dairy. *See also* **Heartburn.**

Acne: foods high in zinc; maple syrup foods with probiotic properties; fermented foods such as yogurt, kimchi, and miso; foods high in omega-3 and GLA fatty acids, such as borage oil, evening primrose oil, fish oil, flaxseed oil, and walnuts; foods high in vitamins A and C; alfalfa sprouts; brewer's yeast; okra; and sea vegetables. Avoid hydrogenated oils. *See also* **Probiotic Foods.**

Allergies, Seasonal; Hay Fever: apples (quercetin); ginger (add to foods or prepare ginger tea); oils high in omega-3 essential fatty acids such as fish oil, flaxseed oil, hemp oil, pumpkin oil, borage oil, and evening primrose oil; and probiotic foods such as Jerusalem artichokes, okra, kimchi, sauerkraut, and miso. Avoid mucus-producing foods such as dairy products, sugar, wheat, and food additives.

Alzheimer's Disease: fiber-rich fruits and vegetables, especially pomegranate juice and bell peppers; healthy fats such as borage oil, fish oil, evening primrose oil, and flaxseed oil; and turmeric.

Anemia, Iron-Deficient: beet greens, blackstrap molasses, kidney beans, liver (always organic and grass-fed if possible), fresh peas, pinto beans, rice bran, lentils, lima beans, mustard greens, spinach.

Antiaging: fruits and vegetables—up to ten servings per day—especially blueberries, blackberries, raspberries, and huckleberries; healthy fats such as borage oil, coconut oil, evening primrose oil, fish oil, and flaxseed oil; antioxidant-rich foods like acai, amla, star fruit, cacao powder, cacao nibs, cactus pear fruit, goji berries, grapes, blue-green algae, bee pollen, reishi mushrooms. Avoid trans fats, processed foods.

Arthritis: *See* **Osteoarthritis** and **Rheumatoid Arthritis.**

Asthma: fresh fruits, vegetables, and whole grains; green smoothies (smoothies made with blended fresh greens, powdered greens, or juice mixed with powdered greens); foods or oils high in omega-3 EFAs such as fish oil, flaxseed oil, and walnuts; foods high in antioxidants; foods high in vitamin C such as bell peppers, berries, citrus fruits, and kiwis; foods high in carotenes such as green, yellow, and orange fruits; vegetables high in carotenoids; foods high in vitamin E, including wheat germ oil, nuts, and seeds; berries, garlic, ginger, onions, radicchio, and turmeric. Avoid all foods that create allergic reactions (consult a health care provider for testing); processed sugar; processed foods, especially those containing white flour, black tea, and coffee.

Atherosclerosis, Prevention: fresh fruits and vegetables, especially dark berries, citrus fruits, and orange and yellow vegetables; fiber-rich foods such as legumes, fruits, and vegetables; healthy fats like cold-pressed organic olive oil, flax oil, fish oil, borage oil, and evening primrose oil; nuts, including almonds, Brazil nuts, hazelnuts, pistachios, pine nuts, sesame seeds, sunflower seeds, and raw walnuts; apple cider vinegar, burdock root, garlic cloves, green tea. Avoid excessive amounts of animal products, fast food, refined carbohydrates, microwaved foods, sugar, and trans fats (hydrogenated oils).

Brain Function and Memory: foods rich in flavonoids, such as blackberries, blueberries, cranberries; eggplant; omega-3 EFAs in fish oil, flaxseed oil, hemp oil, or walnuts; GLAs in borage oil and evening primrose oil.

Breast Cancer, Prevention: foods high in essential fatty acids, such as black currant oil, borage oil, evening primrose oil, fish oil, hemp oil; cruciferous vegetables like broccoli, broccoli sprouts, cabbage, cauliflower; foods high in phytosterols, such as fennel, pumpkin seeds, sunflower seeds; onions, garlic, lentils, guava. Avoid trans fats, microwaved foods, processed food.

Calming Foods: root vegetables, such as carrots, sweet potatoes, and yucca; healthy sweets like fruits and maple syrup; foods high in magnesium and calcium, such as sea vegetables, especially hijiki; foods high in magnesium, like chocolate, blue-green algae, and nuts, especially almonds.

Cancer, Prevention: fresh, organic fruits and vegetables; fiber-rich foods, such as fruits, vegetables, legumes; all berries, especially for stomach cancer; all nuts, especially, almonds, Brazil nuts, pistachios, and walnuts; antioxidant-rich foods like acai, acerola, dark chocolate (preferably mixed with raw cacao), ginger, grapes, persimmons, noni, raddichio, star fruit; foods high in quercetin, such as apples and onions; all types of sprouts, especially alfalfa sprouts and barley sprouts; all types of seaweeds; natto, parsley, mangosteen juice, mushrooms, tea, spinach, sunflower seeds, okra, ginger, and watercress (especially for smokers); cruciferous vegetables such as broccoli, broccoli sprouts, brussels sprouts, and kale. Avoid trans fats; microwaved foods; exposure to substances that create free radicals, such as cigarette smoke, toxic household cleaners, and pesticides.

Candida; Yeast Infection: probiotic foods, yogurt (especially after taking antibiotics), kefir, kimchi. Increase foods and substances that support digestion, such as bitters, water with fresh lemon juice, okra, and foods rich in water-soluble fiber—especially psyllium seeds and pectin-rich foods. Other foods to increase are oregano, oregano oil, coconut oil, coconut milk, and immune-enhancing foods. Mix 1 tablespoon raw, unfiltered apple cider vinegar with 8 ounces water. Add stevia or raw honey, if needed, and aloe vera juice to taste. Avoid alcohol, yeast foods, such as yeast breads, maple syrup, food allergens (check with your health care provider for testing), refined sugar, refined flour. *See also* **Probiotic Foods.**

Canker Sores: Eliminate food allergens (check with your health care provider a for specific testing). *See also* **Herpes.**

Cardiovascular Disease; Heart Disease, Prevention: fruits and vegetables (five or more servings per day), especially apples, garlic, leeks, and onions; raw nuts, olive oil, fish oil, flax oil, borage oil, evening primrose oil, and other omega-3 oils; garbanzo beans, shitake mushrooms; fiber-rich fruits and vegetables, especially eggplant, okra, amaranth greens; whole grains, especially amaranth, buckwheat, and oats. Drink plenty of water, apple juice, and fresh fruit or vegetable juices. Avoid refined foods, including meat and especially salt.

Carpal Tunnel: foods rich in vitamin B6, including brewer's yeast, sunflower seeds, soybeans, walnuts, lentils, other legumes, brown rice, and bananas; foods with anti-inflammatory properties, such as pineapples, pineapple juice, fresh ginger, and turmeric. Avoid processed foods containing tartrazine (FD&C Yellow No. 5). *See also* **Repetitive Strain Injury.**

Cataracts, Prevention: foods with high antioxidant levels, especially berries, broccoli, carrots, leafy greens, fresh fruits, wheat germ oil, wheatgrass juice, yams; foods high in glutathione, such as parsley, fresh fruits, and vegetables. Avoid: fried foods, processed table salt, trans fats.

Celiac Disease; Gluten Intolerance: non-glutenous grains like amaranth, quinoa, rices (brown, red, black, and wild), sorghum, tamari (wheat free), papaya, probiotic foods, kimchi, sauerkraut. Avoid foods containing gluten, wheat, rye, barley, spelt, Kamut, or oats; soy sauce with gluten.

Constipation: fruits; high-fiber foods such as whole grains; water and other non-caffeinated drinks; magnesium-rich foods, such as nuts and raw chocolate; barley juice, flaxseed oil, okra, nopales cactus, plums, prunes, psyllium seeds or husks, raisins, raspberries, raw honey, rhubarb, wheatgrass juice.

Dandruff: Dandruff is usually a sign that your body has too much yeast. Increase garlic, probiotics, borage oil. *See also* **Yeast Infection.**

Depression: foods and oils high in omega-3 essential fatty acids, such as fish oil, flaxseed oil, hemp milk powder, hemp protein, pumpkins or pumpkin seed oil, walnuts, walnut oil; foods high in folate like mustard greens, beans, spinach; ginger, lemon balm, peas. Avoid alcohol, diet sodas, and products containing aspartame, NutraSweet, or Equal.

Detox: *See* **Liver Detox; Kitchari; Mung Bean.**

Diabetes: foods high in quercetin such as onions, apples, evening primrose oil, borage oil, black currant oil, cinnamon, huckleberries, psyllium husks, nuts; fiber-rich fruits and vegetables; foods that regulate blood sugar, such as spirulina, maca, brewer's yeast, egg yolks, seaweed (especially kelp), garlic, sauerkraut, and fiber-rich vegetables; bitter gourd, nopales cactus, aloe vera gel or juice, fenugreek, garbanzo beans, noni juice, cinnamon, garlic, ginger, hijiki, lemon balm tea, stevia. Avoid processed foods, diet sodas, and all products containing artificial sweeteners such as aspartame, NutraSweet, or Equal.

Diarrhea: If an infection is present, diarrhea is often accompanied by a fever. In acute stages, avoid solid foods. Replace water and electrolytes lost during bouts of diarrhea with broths, coconut water, or electrolyte drinks. In acute stages, increase: coconut water, raw honey alone or mixed with water, diluted non-caffeinated fluids, pomegranate juice, mint tea, vegetable broth, vegetable juices. During chronic stage, increase: black currant oil, blueberries, carob powder or chips, kefir, pomegranates, mangoes, raw chocolate or raw cacao; pectin-rich fruits and vegetables, such as apples, nopales cactus, pears, grapefruits, carrots, potatoes, and beets; psyllium seeds or husks. Avoid dairy products except yogurt and kefir, food allergens.

Diverticulitis: alfalfa, aloe vera, green leafy vegetables.

Dry skin: yellow-orange fruits and vegetables such as yellow squashes, mangoes, and papayas; evening primrose oil; omega-3 oils, such as fish oil, flaxseed oil, or coconut oil.

Eczema: borage oil, evening primrose oil, flaxseed oil; all other foods or oils rich in essential fatty acids; kelp; foods high in vitamin C such as red bell peppers, parsley, amla berries; foods high in zinc.

Endometriosis: alfalfa, burdock root, garlic. Avoid alcohol and caffeine.

Eye Health: broccoli, raw cabbage, carrots, cauliflower, green vegetables, squash, sunflower seeds, watercress. *See also* **Macular Degeneration.**

Fibrocystic Breasts: bananas, whole grains, seeds, nuts, brussels sprouts, cauliflower, legumes, fruits, nuts, seeds, yams, wheat germ oil, vegetables; plenty of water and fluids; foods high in fiber; and foods that promote regular bowel movements. Avoid caffeine, chocolate, processed foods.

Flu; Bronchitis; Pneumonia, Prevention: foods that build immunity, such as fresh organic natural foods, fruits and vegetables (such as acerola, amla, kiwi, parsley, lemon, cayenne, orange, rambuton, bell peppers, parika), whole grains, legumes, nuts, and seeds. Avoid foods high in refined sugars, refined carbohydrates. Studies have shown a diet high in fruits and vegetables reduces the risk of pneumonia and bronchitis. During flu, bronchitis, or pneumonia, eat raw pineapple, raw garlic, or cooked radish.

Gallstones: fresh vegetables and fruits; foods high in fiber, including flaxseeds, oat bran, psyllium seeds and husks; foods high in pectin, such as apples, onions, grapefruit. Avoid animal proteins, dairy products; processed foods and sugars.

Gas; Flatulence: Chew on ajwain seeds or make a tea or water with lemon juice and ajwain seeds; anise seeds; fennel.

Glaucoma, Chronic: fresh fruits, vegetables, whole grains, nuts, seeds; foods high in vitamin C, such as citrus fruits, kiwis, bell peppers, blueberries, bilberries; foods containing omega-3 oils, such as flaxseeds, walnuts, fish, hemp seeds, pumpkin seeds, fish oil, flax oil, walnut oil, macadamia nut oil.

Gout: cherries and cherry juice, water, pineapple; foods low in purine, such as eggs, fruit, especially strawberries, apples, grains, milk, pasta, nuts, seeds, olives, parsley, celery, and celery juice. Avoid alcohol, refined carbohydrates, refined sugars, foods high in purine, anchovies, red meat, meat broth, fish meat, organ meats, yeast, moderate purine foods, asparagus, legumes, mushrooms, dried peas, poultry, shellfish, spinach.

Hangover: nopales cactus, coconut water, asparagus, celery, Irish moss, aloe vera, wheatgrass, barley grass.

Hair, Skin, and Nails: seaweed, especially hijiki; parsnips; wheatgrass.

Heartburn; Acid Reflux: unsweetened cranberry juice (sip it); aloe vera leaves or juice; vegetable blend juices including greens, cucumber, lemon, and carrot. Try eating slowly! A study at the University of South Carolina compared people who rushed through a meal in five minutes with those who ate at a leisurely pace of thirty minutes. Those that shoveled down their food had significantly higher incidents of acid reflux than those who slowed down. Avoid onions, tomatoes, coffee.

Hemorrhoids: fruits, legumes, vegetables, whole grains; foods rich in flavonoids, such as blackberries, blueberries, cherries, buckwheat, and citrus foods including peels; foods with lots of fiber; foods with bioflavonoids, such as colorful berries like blueberries, blackberries, and cherries as well as bitter melon. Also be sure to drink plenty of water when suffering from hemorrhoids. Avoid alcohol, processed foods, coffee, spicy foods. *See also* **Varicose Veins**.

Herpes, Prevention of Outbreaks: foods high in lysine, such as baked beans, eggs, meat, milk, cheese, pork; foods high in vitamin C, garlic, and thyme. During a herpes outbreak, dip a cloth in milk and apply for 5 seconds, then take off for 5 seconds. Continue for 5 minutes, and repeat every 3–4 hours. Avoid foods high in arginine like chocolate, peas, nuts, and beer.

High Blood Pressure: foods high in calcium and magnesium; foods high in omega-3 fatty acids, such as fish, flaxseeds, macadamia nuts, pumpkin seeds, walnuts, fish oil, flaxseed oil, hemp oil; celery, garlic, onion, nuts and seeds, green leafy vegetables, seaweed; foods rich in vitamin C such as citrus fruits and bell peppers. Diet and lifestyle have been shown to be very important for reducing blood pressure. Reduce stress and get plenty of exercise. Avoid processed foods, refined sugars and carbohydrates, alcohol, caffeine, and tobacco.

Hypoglycemia: Follow recommendations for diabetes. Increase vegetables, protein, whole grains, healthy fats. Avoid alcohol.

Immune Support: fresh fruits, vegetables, whole grains, legumes, seeds, nuts; adequate but not excessive amounts of protein; foods high in carotenes to support the thymus gland, including yellow and orange vegetables, carrots, yams, red peppers, and tomatoes; cabbage family of vegetables, including broccoli, brussels sprouts, cauliflower, and kale; flavonoid-rich foods; all berries including acai, blackberries, blueberries, radicchio: bee pollen, black currant oil, colostrums, garlic, Jerusalem artichokes, mushrooms, especially shitake and reishi; plenty of water and healthy fluids; yogurt, especially with *Bifidobacterium lactis*; foods rich in magnesium, like raw or dark chocolate, pumpkin seeds, spinach, Swiss chard, sunflower seeds, sesame seeds, halibut, and black beans; foods high in zinc, such as maple syrup, pumpkin; foods high in B vitamins, such as whole grains, leafy greens and legumes, sea vegetables, sesame, milk, dairy, raw cacao. Avoid refined sugars, stress, alcohol, allergy-triggering foods, and caffeine. *See also* **Calming Foods.**

Indigestion: ajwain seeds: drink as a tea, chew on the seeds, or make a concoction with lemon juice. Also helpful are aloe vera, ginger, okra, fennel and fennel seeds, Irish moss, noni, pineapple, and papaya.

Inflammation: ajwain, apples, flaxseeds, turmeric, broccoli, *Brassica* genus, fish oil, cod liver oil, flaxseed oil, blue-green algae, noni, nata, pomegranate, blueberries, acai, pumpkin seeds.

Insomnia: celery, carrot-celery juice; root vegetables such as carrots, parsnips, radicchio, potatoes, and sweet potatoes; foods high in tryptophan; almonds, milk, cashew nuts, cottage cheese, chicken, turkey; foods rich in magnesium, including raw or dark chocolate, pumpkin seeds, spinach, Swiss chard, sunflower seeds, sesame seeds, halibut, and black beans. Avoid caffeinated soft drinks, chocolate, coffee, hot chocolate and tea, refined sugars and refined carbohydrates.

Irritable Bowel Syndrome: fiber-rich fruits and vegetables; fresh raw ginger or fresh raw ginger juice added to other vegetable or fruit drinks. Avoid food allergens, refined sugars, refined carbohydrates.

Intestinal Parasites: Coconut and coconut oil, garlic, oregano, pineapple, propolis, pumpkin seeds, turmeric. Avoid caffeine, alcohol, and refined sugar and foods.

Kidney Stones: plenty of water and fluids, cranberries, fresh cranberry juice. Consume in moderation: low-oxalate fruits and veggies such as berries, brussels sprouts, carrots, green peas, leeks, and nuts such as cashews and peanuts. Avoid foods high in oxalates, such as beet greens, collard greens, rhubarb, spinach, Swiss chard; alcohol, processed foods, refined sugars, excess animal proteins, and trans fats.

Liver Detox: The liver helps to move toxins out of the body and is important for weight loss, as the body releases body fat and toxins stored within that fat. Increase cruciferous veggies like broccoli, broccoli sprouts, brussels sprouts, cabbage, and cauliflower as well as leafy greens, beet greens, dandelion or mustard greens, collard, chard, or watercress; cilantro and parsley; citrus fruits like orange, lemon, or lime; sulfur-rich foods like daikon radishes, eggs, garlic, and onions; burdock root; aloe vera leaves and juice; liver-building foods like fresh cooked artichoke, asparagus, beets, celery, colostrum, sprouts, and nutritional yeast. Drink lots of purified water when supporting or detoxifying the liver. Add lemon to boost your filtered water's liver-cleansing ability.

Longevity: *See* **Antiaging.**

Macular Degeneration: yellow and orange carotenes such as red peppers, kiwi, tomatoes, sweet potatoes, carrots, squash, broccoli; green leafy vegetables such as collard greens, kale, mustard greens, spinach and turnip greens; legumes, flavonoid-rich berries, especially blueberries, bilberries, blackberries, and cherries. Avoid refined foods, trans fats, microwaved foods.

Menopause: foods high in phytoestrogens, including soybeans, tofu, miso, flaxseeds, nuts, whole grains, apples, celery, fennel, fenugreek, parsley, and alfalfa; cruciferous vegetables, such as broccoli, brussels sprouts, cabbages, collards, kale, mustard and turnip greens; foods that support the liver, like aloe vera gel or juice, daikon; bee pollen

Migraine: Eat to keep blood sugar levels steady. Avoid aged cheeses, beer, chicken liver, chocolate, food additives, wine, brewer's yeast.

Multiple Sclerosis: borage oil, evening primrose oil, fish, fish oil, flaxseed oil, macadamia nut oil, walnuts, pumpkin seeds. Avoid food allergens.

Muscle Cramps: foods rich in magnesium, like raw or dark chocolate, pumpkin seeds, spinach, Swiss chard, sunflower seeds, sesame seeds, halibut, and black beans.

Osteoarthritis: alfalfa, asparagus, barley grass; berries such as blueberries, blackberries; borage seed oil for pain control; cruciferous vegetables such as brussels sprouts, cabbage; cherries, daikon, evening primrose oil; omega-3 oils like fish oil, flaxseed oil, and hemp oil; apples, cucumbers, noni, garlic, ginger, onions, parsnips, pumpkin seeds, strawberries, turmeric, wheatgrass. Avoid processed foods and vegetables from the nightshade family such as tomatoes, potatoes, eggplant, peppers.

Osteoporosis: cruciferous vegetables from the cabbage family, including broccoli, brussels sprouts, collards, kale, mustard greens; alfalfa; borage oil and evening primrose oil; celery, edamame, green tea, maca, natto, onions, soybeans, Swiss chard, tofu. Avoid excess protein, refined salt, soft drinks or carbonated drinks containing phosphates, refined sugar.

Pregnancy, Health During: fruits and vegetables (five or more servings per day); pineapple, dried or fresh papaya for indigestion, mango, star fruit, cucumber, watermelon, cantaloupe, honeydew melon; amaranth, ginger, fennel, millet for morning sickness, alfalfa, wheat germ; dark leafy greens; grass-fed beef, chicken; cheese, yogurt; beets, lentils, spinach, kale, parsnips, fenugreek, fennel, fennel seed tea for lactation; walnuts, filberts.

Premenstrual Syndrome, PMS: daikon radishes; evening primrose oil; edamame, fennel, yams, leafy green vegetables, spinach and legumes; miso, tofu, soybeans, seaweed, tempeh; yogurt, whole milk; sunflower seeds, chickpeas, quinoa, almonds, pecans, avocado; buckwheat, millet; molasses, cacao powder, cacao nibs, dark chocolate. Avoid animal products, caffeine, refined salt.

Probiotic Foods: Jerusalem artichokes, coconut water, yogurt, miso, okra, kimchi, sauerkraut, tempeh, buttermilk, kombucha.

Prostate Enlargement; Prostate Cancer, Prevention: unprocessed foods, whole grains, legumes, fruits, nuts, and vegetables; foods containing lycopene, especially tomatoes, tomato sauce, guava, watermelon, berries; spinach, kale, mango; pumpkin seeds, sunflower seeds, Brazil nuts; maple syrup; saw palmetto berries, whole or extract; minimally processed tofu or soybeans; garlic. Avoid alcohol, especially beer; caffeine, meat, milk, foods containing pesticides, sugar.

Psoriasis: foods high in omega-3 fatty acids, such as cold-water fish like salmon, mackerel, herring, and halibut; fish oil, flaxseed oil, pumpkin seed oil. Avoid alcohol, gluten, animal fats, meat, dairy products, sugar.

Radiation: foods that reduce the stress of exposure to radiation from mobile phones, microwaves, computers, air travel, x-rays and cancer therapies are maitake mushrooms, oranges, noni, mangosteen, parsley, acai.

Repetitive Strain Injury (RSI); Carpal Tunnel: foods with anti-inflammatory properties; flaxseed oil, fresh ground flaxseed, turmeric, horseradish, ginger.

Rheumatoid Arthritis: fresh fruits and vegetables, vegetarian or fish diet (has been shown to be beneficial in the treatment of inflammatory conditions such as rheumatoid arthritis, for several reasons including increasing the amount of fresh fruit and vegetables); antioxidant-rich foods, including acai, acerola, star fruit; carotene-rich foods; yellow and green vegetables, including carrots, cabbage family vegetables, squash, and yams; flavonoid-rich foods such as blueberries, blackberries, cherries, cranberries, raspberries, and strawberries; foods high in vitamin C; wheat germ oil; Brazil nuts; foods high in molybdenum, especially adzuki beans as well as other legumes, brewer's yeast, cauliflower, and spinach; fresh, lightly cooked ginger; horseradish; pineapple; pumpkin seeds; turmeric; spleen-strengthening foods like parsley, garlic, daikon and other radishes, turnips, barley grass, and adzuki beans; foods rich in omega-3 fatty acids such as cold-water fish such as halibut, salmon, and sardines; pharmaceutical grade fish oil. Replace all fats with olive oil, but do not heat above 200°F. Cook with a cooking spray or minute amounts of oil, and after cooking add olive oil or other cold-pressing oils such as black currant oil, borage oil, flaxseed oil, evening primrose oil. Avoid food allergens (see a doctor for testing), most common allergenic foods include beef, corn, coffee, dairy products, milk, nightshade family foods (eggplants, peppers, potatoes, tobacco, and tomatoes).

Ulcers; Peptic Ulcer Disease: foods high in fiber; foods that will fight *H. pylori*, such as garlic, cayenne pepper, turmeric; foods high in vitamin C; foods high in sulforaphane such as cruciferous vegetables including broccoli, cabbage, and cauliflower; aloe vera (whole leaf, gel, or juice), cranberries, cranberry juice, bananas, Irish moss, and Manuka honey. Avoid food allergens (check with your health care provider for allergy testing), especially milk.

Urinary Tract Infection: unsweetened cranberry juice, unsweetened blueberry juice, concentrated cranberry extract in a pill form;

filtered water, herbal teas; fresh fruit and vegetable juices, diluted with half water. Avoid alcohol, caffeine, concentrated fruit juices, drinks sweetened with high fructose corn syrup, soft drinks.

Varicose Veins: Diet should be high in fiber and rich in fruits, vegetables, legumes, and whole grains. Flavonoid rich foods such as blackberries, blueberries, cherries; pith or white part of the skin of citrus fruits such as lemons, kumquats, grapefruit, and oranges; buckwheat tea; nuts, especially those high in arginine, such as almonds, hazelnuts, peanuts, sunflower seeds, and walnuts; foods that increase fibrinolytic action of the blood, including cayenne pepper, garlic, ginger, natto, onion; fresh pineapple, grape juice, and grape seeds.

Vitamins and Minerals: *See table on pp. 151–52.*

Weight Loss: black or green tea, foods rich in water-soluble fibers such as psyllium seeds, chia, fenugreek seeds, pectin, and whole seaweed, especially arame, hijiki, powdered seaweed fibers; agar, carrageen: stevia, cayenne; purified water, purified water with apple cider vinegar (8 ounces water for 1 tablespoon apple cider vinegar, stevia optional); blue-green algae, bok choy, cabbage; celery and celery juice, soup, chicken broth, vegetable broth; garlic, ginger, peas, radicchio, summer squashes, and zucchini. *See also* **Liver Detox.**

Workout Recovery: celery and/or carrot juice, coconut water, prunes, raisins; high-quality proteins, especially minimally processed protein powders made from whey or vegetable proteins (mix with water or blend into a smoothie); prunes, chestnuts, ginger, oregano, oil of oregano for sore muscles. Avoid all processed foods, especially processed carbohydrates, refined sugars.

Vitamins

Most multivitamin supplements contain vitamins that have been chemically isolated in a laboratory. When a vitamin's structure is recreated in a lab, it may not be as effective as a vitamin contained in an original food source. Vitamins that come from whole food sources work synergistically with other vitamins, minerals, and phytonutrients contained within its original food source. For example, vitamin C created in a lab has many benefits, yet a higher quality can be obtained from foods that are extremely high in vitamin C, such as amla and acerola berries. These fruits can be dried and used in powder, paste, or tablet form. Many ancient cultures made supplements from whole foods. Dehydrating or concentrating nutrient-dense foods such as seaweed, berries, barley grass, and alfalfa has many benefits. These whole foods contain many vitamins, minerals, and phytonutrients that work as a team and may be more easily utilized by the body as a complete package. In addition, they may have other phytochemical compounds that have not yet been discovered. Scientists are constantly discovering new chemical compounds in plants that have health benefits for humans. Concentrated whole foods can be stored for longer periods of time than fresh whole foods and can be consumed therapeutically to treat various health conditions.

Vitamins and Minerals in Brief and Key Terms for Reading this Guide

Vitamins and minerals are natural substances found in plants and animals that keep us healthy and support many bodily functions.

Vitamin A; Retinol; Beta-Carotene	fights infection; healthy vision and skin; bone growth; cell division
Vitamin B$_1$; Thiamine	energy release; growth; healthy nervous system
Vitamin B$_2$; Riboflavin	energy release; growth; healthy eyes, skin, hair, and nails; formation of red blood cells
Vitamin B$_3$; Niacin	manufactures hormones; healthy eyes, skin, hair, and nails
Vitamin B$_5$; Pantothenic Acid	adrenal function; antistress
Vitamin B6; Pyridoxine	protein metabolism; growth; infection protection; forms red blood cells and neurotransmitters; maintains hormone balance; healthy immune function
Vitamin B$_{12}$	forms red blood cells; protects nerves; DNA formation
Biotin	metabolism; fat synthesis; waste excretion
Vitamin C	makes collagen; antioxidant; aids in iron absorption; essential for formation, growth, and repair of bones and skin
Calcium	healthy bones and teeth; nerve impulses; muscle contraction
Choline	metabolism
Copper	blood and bone formation

Vitamin D	calcium absorption; immune function
Vitamin E	antioxidant
Folate; Folic Acid	fertility; health during pregnancy; essential for healthy cell formation
Iodine	thyroid hormones; metabolism; growth; reproduction
Iron	forms red blood cells; circulation
Vitamin K	protein creation for blood clotting; bone health
Magnesium	enzymes activation; energy production; cellular reproduction; muscle relaxation
Manganese	antioxidant; energy production
Molybdenum	iron usage; DNA metabolism
Phosphorus	strong teeth and bones
Potassium	fluid and pH level regulation; blood pressure regulation
Selenium	antioxidant
Sodium	fluid regulation
Zinc	immune function; tissue formation

Glossary

Acetogenins: Enormously more powerful than many chemotherapy drugs like Adriamycin (some estimates are one million to one billion times more powerful), acetogenins don't damage the physical body like chemotherapy drugs do. Acetogenins are found in trees and plants and most especially in the paw-paw tree.

Acetylcholine; ACh: This neurotransmitter plays a role in muscle movement and heart regulation. ACh is believed to play a role in learning, memory, and mood. A shortage of ACh has been associated with Alzheimer's disease.

Adaptogen: A plant-derived agent that increases the human body's ability to deal with stress, adaptogens are not toxic when taken in reasonable quantities. They benefit the body as a whole, and they help create balance or "normalization" throughout the body.

Anthocyanadins: Plant pigments that are like anthocyanins, but differ in chemical structure. *See also* **anthocyanins**.

Anthocyanins: Water-soluble plant pigments that give fruits and vegetables their red, blue, and purple colors, anthocyanins are flavonoids with potent antioxidant abilities. Research has shown anthocyanins can protect against cancer, aging, inflammation, diabetes, bacterial infections, and neurological diseases.

Ayurveda: The ancient Indian science based on Vedic texts, *Ayurveda* literally means "science of life." In regards to diet, Ayurvedic philosophy considers each person as having a mind/body/spirit blueprint, a kind of elemental fingerprint, called a *dosha*. Ayurveda wisely advises people to eat based on their unique blueprint to create balance.

Beta-glucans: Phytochemicals present in barley, oats, and shitake mushrooms, beta-glucans have immune-enhancing properties and help improve glucose tolerance while lowering insulin output.

Beta-sitosterols: Found in pecans, avocados, and pumpkin seeds, beta-sitosterol has a chemical structure similar to cholesterol. When used in conjunction with other similar phytosterols, it has been shown to reduce levels of unhealthy cholesterol.

Brassica: The Brassica genus of cruciferous vegetables includes broccoli, bok choy, and cauliflower.

Catechins: Catechins are antioxidant phytochemicals, abundant in tea and chocolate. Various catechins demonstrate a wide range of healthful benefits including antibiotic properties and cardio-protective effects. Catechins in green tea may suppress the growth of tumors and the spread of cancer.

Coenzyme Q10; CoQ10: CoQ10 is an oil-soluble, vitamin-like substance responsible for generating energy in the body through a process called ATP. Organs with high energy requirements like the heart and liver have the highest content of CoQ10 and the highest nutritional need for it. CoQ10 is present in spinach and other foods.

FDA: The Food and Drug Administration.

Glucosinolates: Glucosinolates are a class of organic compounds found in cruciferous vegetables. Studies suggest that they have anticancer properties, helping the body to eliminate carcinogens.

Macrobiotic Diet: Macrobiotics encourage living within the natural order of life. The diet itself consists of a whole foods pesco-vegetarian diet (a diet that includes fish, but no other red meat, poultry, or animal products). Guidelines recommend that 50–60 percent of the diet be whole grains, 25–30 percent vegetables, 5–10 percent miso and bean soups, and 5–10 perecent legumes and sea vegetables.

Oleic Acid: An omega-9 monounsaturated fat found in animal and plant sources, oleic acid is considered a healthy fat. Abundant in olive oil and acai, it has been shown to help prevent heart disease and promote the production of antioxidants.

Polyacetylenes: Polyacetylenes are compounds found in root vegetables with possible chemo-protective and anticarcinogenic effects.

Phytoestrogens: Present in foods such as flax and soybeans, phytoestrogens are compounds that mimic the hormone estrogen, and some evidence suggests that they have a balancing effect on estrogen. If there is too much estrogen, which can be a risk factor for breast and ovarian cancer, phytoestrogens may help block the absorption of excess estrogen in the body. On the other hand, phytoestrogens may help boost estrogenic activity in women whose estrogen levels are low. There is some fear that phytoestrogens may be detrimental for women who suffer from cancers associated with excessive levels of estrogen. Even with mixed evidence, the role of phytoestrogens in the diet can have many benefits.

Phytosterols: Similar to cholesterol and naturally occurring in plants, phytosterols block cholesterol absorption and maintain the integrity of cell membranes. The FDA has approved a claim that phytosterols may reduce the risk of heart disease.

Raw Food Diet: A raw food diet consists of foods not heated above 98°F. Cooking often destroys more than 75 percent of food's vitamins, enzymes, and phytonutrients, so increasing the amount of raw, plant-based foods ingested can significantly boost nutritional intake. Reported benefits of a raw food diet are increased energy, improved digestion, weight loss, and reduced risk for many degenerative diseases.

Resveratrol: A polyphenolic compound found in red wine, grapes, peanuts, and some berries. In animal studies, it has demonstrated anti-inflammatory, anticancer, cardio-protective, and blood sugar-stabilizing effects. It has been reported to extend the life of insects and mice fed a high-calorie diet.

Saponins: A class of compounds found in plants, saponins have been shown to have beneficial effects on blood cholesterol levels, bone health, and immune system health while also preventing cancer.

Sulforaphane: Present in cruciferous vegetables, sulforaphane is a substance that has anticancer properties and may help boost immunity.

Superoxide Dismutase, SOD: An antioxidant enzyme instrumental in neutralizing damaging free radicals, thereby slowing cellular deterioration, cell mutation, tumor growth as well as the ordinary oxidative stress associated with aging. SOD is present in green vegetables, especially wheatgrass, barley grass, and parsley.

Tannins: Tannins are plant polyphenols with an astringent flavor and have anti-inflammatory and potential antiviral, antibacterial, and anticancer effects.

Theobromine: Theobromine is a bitter alkaloid and mild stimulant found in the cacao plant, kola nut, and acai berry.

Tocitrienols: This group of related compounds has vitamin E activity and is also known for fat-soluble antioxidants. Tocitrienols make up four of vitamin E's eight forms.

Tocopherols: Tocopherols are fat-soluble antioxidants that have vitamin E activity. Vitamin E exists in eight forms, four of which are tocopherols.

Traditional Chinese Medicine: Traditional Chinese medicine utilizes a complex diagnostic system that takes practitioners many years to learn. An initial analysis of imbalances within a patient is determined through physical observation, reportage of current symptoms as well as diet and lifestyle, and often a pulse diagnosis. A treatment plan and dietary recommendations are then formulated based on these diagnoses.

Triglycerides: Fatty acids that can be measured in the blood stream. High levels of triglycerides are associated with greater risk of stroke and heart disease.

Tryptophan: An essential amino acid that must be obtained from food, tryptophan is best known for its role as a chemical precursor to serotonin, the feel-good neurotransmitter. Plentiful sources of tryptophan are sesame, pumpkin and sunflower seeds, poultry—especially turkey—and milk.

USRDA: Recommended daily intake of specific vitamins, minerals, and macronutrients for a healthy person as established by the Food and Nutrition Board of the National Academy of Sciences. The RDA does not take into account the quality nor form of the vitamin, mineral, or macronutrient ingested, nor the differences between individuals. For example, a pregnant woman has much different nutritional needs than a woman who is not pregnant.

Vegan Diet: The vegan diet is the same as a vegetarian diet, but without dairy products. The Physicians Committee for Responsible Medicine advocates a vegan diet.

Vegetarian Diet: Vegetarians do not consume animal flesh, although some vegetarians consume eggs and/or dairy products. Vegetarian diets have been studied scientifically and have been shown to help with weight loss, decreased risk of cardiovascular disease, lowering cholesterol and blood pressure levels, decreased rates of type 2 diabetes, and various types of cancers.

Weston A. Price Foundation: In the 1920s, Weston Price had become dismayed with the dental health of his American patients and began studying eating habits of people without modern industrialized food. The Weston A. Price Foundation has chapters around the world and endorses a nonvegetarian diet based on traditional whole foods, naturally raised, grass-fed meats, and raw dairy products. Processed foods, including nontraditional soy products, are shunned.

Online Shopping and Resource Guide

www.aaaomonline.org: Resource on traditional Chinese medicine, including information on finding a practitioner.

www.amerveg.com: Provides information and kits on how to become a vegetarian.

www.arizonacactusranch.com: Source for prickly pear cactus nectar foods, information, and recipes.

www.ayurfoods.com: AyurFoods makes Dr. Jay Apte's ready-to-cook kitchari for busy people.

www.ayurveda-nama.org: Provides information on Ayurveda and resources for finding an Ayurvedic practitioner.

www.banyanbotanicals.com: Chyavanprash and other organic Indian spices are available at this Web site.

www.bobsredmill.com: Excellent source for organic grains, beans, seeds, cereals, and flours.

www.compassionatecooks.com: Recommended Web site for following a vegan diet.

www.foodnews.org: Information on how to reduce exposure to pesticides. Foodnews.org publishes the Dirty Dozen—the twelve fruits and vegetables most contaminated by pesticides—as well as the Clean Fifteen—the fifteen least contaminated nonorganic fruits and vegetables. Download the iPhone app or PDF to carry with you when you shop.

www.goveg.com: Provides information and kits on how to become a vegetarian.

www.kushiinstitute.org: Macrobiotic educational programs and information.

www.larabar.com: Snack bars made of raw whole foods, with three to five fruits and nuts and sweetened with dates. Vitamin- and fiber-rich!

www.loaj.com: Provides information on Ayurveda and resources for finding an Ayurvedic practitioner.

www.macrobiotics.co.uk: Useful tips on following a macrobiotic diet.

www.organicindia.com: Recommended for tulsi teas as well as powerful food herbs like amalki, tulsi, and turmeric.

www.organicpastures.com: Provides information on raw milk and other raw dairy products. They will ship raw dairy products within California.

www.pcrm.org: The Physicians Committee for Responsible Medicine provides information on the New Four Food Groups, as well as published research on the benefits of a vegan diet.

www.rawvitamins.com: Offers high-quality, whole food vitamin supplements.

www.saltworks.us: Source for gourmet sea salt from around the world as well as information on the health benefits of sea salt.

www.southrivermiso.com: Manufacturer of high-quality artisan misos made with sea salt.

www.sproutpeople.com: This site teaches how to make your own sprouts and is also a source for seeds and sprouting equipment.

www.standardprocess.com: Produces high-quality, whole food vitamin supplements and a minimally processed whey protein powder, Whey Pro Complete.

www.sunfood.com: Incredible source of pure, unprocessed foods from around the world. David Wolfe heads Sun Foods and is known for his meticulous procurement of incredibly high-quality raw foods like Wild Jungle Peanuts, noni powder, pure raw chocolate, and aloe leaves.

www.teffco.com: Source for gluten-free teff grain and teff flour grown in Idaho.

www.timpanogosnursery.com: Source for ordering live goji berry and stevia plants and seeds as well as information on how to grow these super foods in your own backyard.

www.truefoodnow.org: Information on food safety for consumers—how to avoid GE (genetically modified) foods as well as food labeling, irradiation, rbGH, factory farms, and fish farming.

www.westonaprice.org: Provides information on the Weston A. Price Foundation and this dietary philosophy.

Bibliography

Balch, Phyllis A. *Prescription for Nutritional Healing*. 4th ed., New York: Avery, 2006.

Colbin, Annemarie. *Food and Healing*. New York: Ballantine Books, 1986.

Cornbleet, Jennifer. *Raw Food Made Easy for One or Two People*. Summertown, TN: The Book Publishing Company, 2005.

Gagne, Steve. *Food Energetics: The Spiritual, Emotional and Nutritional Power of What We Eat*. Rochester, VT: Healing Arts Press, 2008.

Grotto, David, RD, LDN. *101 Foods That Could Save Your Life*. New York: Bantam Dell, 2007.

Haas, Elson M., and Buck Levin. *Staying Healthy with Nutrition, 21st-Century Edition: The Complete Guide to Diet & Nutritional Medicine*. Berkeley: Celestial Arts, 2006.

Hospodar, Miriam Kasin. *Heaven's Banquet: Vegetarian Cooking for Lifelong Health the Ayurveda Way*. New York: Plume, 2001.

La Puma, John, MD, and Rebecca Powell Marx. *Chef MD's Big Book of Culinary Medicine*. New York: Crown Publishing, 2008.

Lad, Vasant, and David Frawley. *Yoga of Herbs: An Ayurvedic Guide to Herbal Medicine*. Twin Lakes, WI: Lotus Press, 2001.

McKeith, Gillian. *Living Food for Health: 12 Natural Superfoods to Transform Your Health*. Laguna Beach, CA: Basic Health Publications, 2005.

Miller, Daphne, MD. *The Jungle Effect: A Doctor Discovers the Healthiest Diets from Around the World—Why They Work and How to Bring Them Home.* New York: Collins Living, 2008.

Minich, Deanna M. *Chakra Foods for Optimum Health: A Guide to the Foods that Can Improve Your Energy, Inspire Creative Changes, Open Your Heart, and Heal Body, Mind, and Spirit.* San Francisco: Conari Press, 2009.

Morningstar, Amadea, and Urmila Desai. *The Ayurvedic Cookbook.* Twin Lakes, WI: Lotus Press,1990.

Pitchford, Paul. *Healing with Whole Foods: Asian Traditions and Modern Nutrition.* 3rd ed. Berkeley: North Atlantic Books, 2002.

Planck, Nina. *Real Food: What to Eat and Why.* New York: Bloomsbury, 2007.

Polunin, Miriam. *Healing Foods.* New York: DK Publishing Inc., 1997.

Rose, Natalia. *The Raw Food Detox Diet: The Five-Step Plan for Vibrant Health and Maximum Weight Loss.* San Francisco: Collins Living, 2006.

———. *Raw Food, Life Force Energy.* San Francisco: Collins Living, 2007.

Smith Jones, Susan. *The Healing Power of Nature Foods: 50 Revitalizing SuperFoods and Lifestyle Choices that Promote Vibrant Health.* Carlsbad: Hay House, 2007.

Swanson, Heidi. *Super Natural Cooking: Five Ways to Incorporate Whole and Natural Ingredients into Your Cooking.* Berkeley: Celestial Arts, 2007.

Ukra, Mark, and Sharyn Kolberg. *The Ultimate Tea Diet.* San Francisco: Collins Living, 2007.

Yeager, Selene, and the Editors of Prevention. *The Doctors Book of Food Remedies.* Revised ed. Emmaus, PA: Rodale, 2008.

About the Author

Elise Marie Collins is a yoga teacher, writer, and spiritual counselor. A graduate of both the University of California at Berkeley and the Berkeley Psychic Institute, Elise loves communicating about health and the healing arts. She has written for *Yoga Journal, Psychic Reader,* and other alternative health magazines and is the author of *Chakra Tonics: Essential Elixirs for the Mind, Body, and Spirit* (Conari 2006). She lives in San Francisco. Visit her on line at: *www.chakratonics.com.*

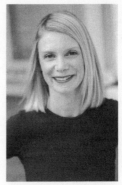

Photograph by Andrea Wyner

To Our Readers

Conari Press, an imprint of Red Wheel/Weiser, publishes books on topics ranging from spirituality, personal growth, and relationships to women's issues, parenting, and social issues. Our mission is to publish quality books that will make a difference in people's lives—how we feel about ourselves and how we relate to one another. We value integrity, compassion, and receptivity, both in the books we publish and in the way we do business.

Our readers are our most important resource, and we value your input, suggestions, and ideas about what you would like to see published. Please feel free to contact us to request our latest book catalog or to be added to our mailing list.

Conari Press
An imprint of Red Wheel/Weiser, LLC
500 Third Street, Suite 230
San Francisco, CA 94107
www.redwheelweiser.com